DATE DUE

Children Surviving Persecution

An International Study of Trauma and Healing

Edited by
Judith S. Kestenberg
and
Charlotte Kahn

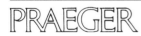

Westport, Connecticut
London

Library of Congress Cataloging-in-Publication Data

Children surviving persecution : an international study of trauma and
  healing / edited by Judith S. Kestenberg and Charlotte Kahn.
      p.   cm.
    Includes bibliographical references and index.
    ISBN 0–275–96261–X (alk. paper)
      1. Holocaust survivors—Mental health.   2. Jewish children in the
  Holocaust.   3. Holocaust, Jewish (1939–1945)—Psychological aspects.
  4. Post-traumatic stress disorder—Age factors.   5. Children of
  Holocaust survivors—Mental health.   6. National socialism—
  Psychological aspects.   7. Stress in children—Longitudinal
  studies.   I. Kestenberg, Judith S.   II. Kahn, Charlotte, 1928–   .
  RC451.4.H62C455   1998
  616.85'21—dc21   98–11124

British Library Cataloguing in Publication Data is available.

Library of Congress Catalog Card Number: 98–11124
ISBN: 0–275–96261–X

First published in 1998

Praeger Publishers, 88 Post Road West, Westport, CT 06881
An imprint of Greenwood Publishing Group, Inc.

Printed in the United States of America

The paper used in this book complies with the
Permanent Paper Standard issued by the National
Information Standards Organization (Z39.48–1984).

10 9 8 7 6 5 4 3 2 1

Copyright Acknowledgments

Grateful acknowledgment is given for permission to quote from the following sources:

Unpublished poem by Eva Löwenthal (1952); "Recurrent Nightmare," by Irene Hizme; Else
Lasker-Schüler, "Das Weltende," in *Sämtliche Gedichte*, ed. Friedhelm Kemp (München: Kösel, 1977).

Every reasonable effort has been made to trace the owners of copyright materials in this
book, but in some instances this has proven impossible. The author and publisher will be
glad to receive information leading to more complete acknowledgments in subsequent print-
ings of the book and in the meantime extend their apologies for any omissions.

Contents

Preface

Charlotte Kahn

Das Weltende
Es ist ein Weinen in der Welt
Als ob der liebe Gott gestorben wär
Und der bleierne Schatten, der nieder fällt,
Lastet grabensschwer.

The End of the World
There is a crying in the world
As if the good God were dead,
And the descending, leaden shadow
Like a tomb, oppressing.

—Else Lasker-Schüler[1]

In this century, few families have escaped the effects of social trauma: Most contain at least one member affected by war or revolution, forced or voluntary relocation, discrimination and ostracism, political harassment, and even torture. The forms and intensity of these experiences have varied, but all have had profound effects on individuals and families, even the milder versions of persistent racism and xenophobia throughout the world, as well as the "red-baiting" of political dissidents in the United States in the 1950s. In an era of continuing eruptions of national, racial, and ethnic violence across the globe, an international perspective, afforded by contributors from nine countries, may add to the understanding of long-term effects of trauma on psychological development.

The prototypical experience of social trauma is the organized persecution of the Holocaust. A study of the aftermath of those shattering events may provide some understanding of how to help surviving victims of other organized persecution, civil violence, and strife. Some contributors to this volume have gleaned their insights into social trauma by living through World War II, and all have studied the responses of the children of the Holocaust— Jewish and non-Jewish, German and non-German. Some engage in a search for meaning; others grapple with the sequelae of trauma as the "unmasking of the illusion of safety."[2] Their conclusions are based on a wealth of interview information and occasionally on clinical material, some of which is presented as evidence, albeit often in the form of brief vignettes. This is consistent with the practice of qualitative research, in which certain subliminal psychological dynamics may be explored in a smaller number of intensive case studies that then serve as paradigms, valued for the validity of their data at least as much as surveys of a much larger population.

In order to maintain easy readability, the aggregate of the available diagnostic data is not presented in statistical form in these chapters. However, clear diagnostic criteria for posttraumatic stress disorder (PTSD) do exist.[3] The disorder is pervasive, characterological, and indicates significant ego impairment. PTSD reactions are quite different from such symptoms as agoraphobia, for example, which is associated with panic disorder. Differences in the symptoms may well be reflective of the severity of the effects of trauma, and a cluster of distinguishing symptoms may be indicative of an impairment of the body or psychological ego relative to the degrees of posttraumatic stress. PTSD may manifest in alterations in mood regulation, hypermnesia (intensified, detailed recall) or amnesia for the traumatic events (including degrees of dissociation or depersonalization) and rumination. In relation to traumatized persons' sense of themselves, feelings of shame and guilt as well as a sense of being different may prevail. Trauma victims may attribute great power to others, seek safety in isolation, or they may search for a rescuer.[4]

Several of the contributors and the editors of this book are themselves survivors of the Holocaust. They have chosen the mental health professions and pedagogy as their vocations—in one instance the law. Kestenberg, Kahn, and the chapter authors combine personal history with psychological insights. They write personally and from the heart.

It was Judith S. Kestenberg's good fortune to arrive in the United States before the outbreak of World War II. Here she devoted her professional life in psychiatry and psychoanalysis to children: children's development, children's movement, and the effects of the organized persecution of children. To document the persecution of children, Dr. Judith S. Kestenberg, director of the Child Development Research organization, established the International Study of Organized Persecution of Children (ISOPC) in 1981, in collaboration with her husband, the late Milton Kestenberg, an attorney and an expert on reparations to Holocaust survivors. To date, under the auspices of the ISOPC, 1,500 child survivors of World War II and the Holocaust have been interviewed by mental health professionals, with anonymity guaranteed, in Eastern and Western Europe, the United States, Israel, Argentina, Australia, and South Africa.

Charlotte Kahn spent the first ten years of her life in Germany, half of this time under Nazi rule. The psychological effects of discrimination and social trauma, as well as of relocation and immigration, have been her personal concerns. As a psychoanalyst and family therapist, these interests have informed her work with patients and students. She joined the ISOPC in 1988 and has conducted an independent investigation of the experiences of East and West Germans who grew up during the Nazi regime. Dr. Kestenberg encouraged her in this pursuit and offered many practical suggestions.

The adult memories of traumatic childhood experiences, recounted in this volume, are accompanied by discussions of their lasting scars and the various mechanisms used to cope with these in the postwar world. These accounts are distinguished by the fact that they are by and about individuals who grew up in *un*exceptional Christian and Jewish families: neither those of high-level Nazis, nor of prominent Jewish scholars or leaders; neither those of resistance fighters, nor of rescuers.

Although considerable overlap was unavoidable, the book has been divided into two parts, each preceded by a brief introduction by Charlotte Kahn. In the first part, *Psychohistorical Perspectives*, sociohistorical aspects and the uniqueness of the Holocaust will be discussed, as well as the Holocaust as a model of persecution with its continuing impact on subsequent generations. To frame, enrich, and provide an expanded context for the biographical and psychological material in this volume, a psychohistorical overview of centuries-long discrimination against Jews has been included (see chapter 1.) The perspectives of the historical context generally, and the evolution of antisemitism specifically, will be discussed, and the psychological and legal issues complicating survivors' attempts to qualify for indemnification will be delineated. The second part, *Children's Responses to Persecution*, will include essays by child survivors from Germany, Holland, Poland, Yugoslavia, and Sweden, in addition to chapters by interviewers of Jewish child survivors and of Germans who grew up under Nazism. The "Afterword" will focus on general trauma responses at various developmental ages, the impact of persecution-derived trauma, and the specific importance of family and other social support systems in times of extreme stress.

It is our intention to present the contributors' accounts as paradigmatic events that might illuminate all manner of traumatic experience—social, sexual, war, physical, and psychological torture. It is the editors' hope that the information in this volume will be of help to survivors and their families, as well as the volunteers and professionals who will come to their aid.

We wish to thank the many survivors who agreed to record their experiences in interviews, who honored us by entrusting us with their feelings of deep pain and loss. Their life stories enlivened our personal memories, their mourning helped us grow beyond ours, and their experiences deepened our understanding of the chapter authors' contributions.

We also acknowledge the assistance of Maria Morrocu Cefalu and Graziella Morrocu, who transcribed the contributors' chapters; Gerald Kahn, who frequently rendered computer first aid; and Jonathan Kahn, who read the chapters and, with an unfailing logic and impeccable writing style, made invaluable contributions.

NOTES

1. Else Lasker-Schüler, "Das Weltende," in *Sämtliche Gedichte (Collected Works)*, ed. Friedhelm Kemp (München: Kösel, 1977), 88, translated here by Charlotte Kahn.

2. Michael Hughes, M.D., "Psychic Trauma: Symptom Formation, Treatment, and Forensic Implications." Paper presented at the Symposium: Psychic Trauma—Clinical and Forensic Issues, American Psychological Association, 105th Annual Convention, August 15–19, 1997.

3. American Psychiatric Association, *Diagnostic and Statistical Manual of Mental Disorders*, 4th ed. (Washington, D.C.: American Psychiatric Association, 1994), 428–29.

4. Judith Lewis Herman, *Trauma and Recovery* (New York: Basic Books, 1992).

Introduction

Charlotte Kahn

Prejudice and contempt, cloaked in the pretense of religious or political conviction, . . . have nearly destroyed us in the past. They plague us still. . . . These obsessions cripple both those who are hated and . . . those who hate, robbing both of what they might become.[1]
—President William Clinton

Rain dances, sacrifices, and prayers attest to humankind's attempts to avert disaster. These organized community practices are evidence not only of credence in supernatural powers (often anthropomorphized), but also of belief in the human power to influence deities and nature. Both are expressions of faith in omnipotence: one vested in outside forces and the other a grandiosity attributed unconsciously to ourselves. These convictions protect against feelings of helplessness in the face of the awesome, inexplicable dangers that have threatened men and women. When a drought is averted, when the storm spares the fisherman, when a child survives a disease, women and men are grateful; they may offer thanks. Sometimes a volcanic eruption destroys a community, a fire consumes the forest, or a flood takes its toll. Like children who need to believe in the goodness of their parents and their parents' ability to protect them, many adults attribute destructive events to a supernatural power's displeasure—even anger—with human deficiencies and badness. They redouble their efforts to please the deities with better behavior, more dances, sacrifices, and prayers. They continue their belief in a benevolent power, and upon themselves they heap guilt—which promises illusionary control over future disasters by remorse and appeasement.

Lamentably, many disasters are man-made. In modern times, wars, torture, and persecution exact at least as great a toll as do most natural disasters.

In the twentieth century, wars on every continent of the earth have killed civilians as well as soldiers; persecutors have tortured children and adult members of racial, ethnic, political, and religious groups; terrorists have murdered unsuspecting citizens with explosives on airplanes, buses, and in public buildings; and in schools, pupils have murdered teachers as well as each other. But in the history of institutionalized, violent persecution (amplified by impulsive deeds) the Holocaust is unique in its inhumane level of sadism and in the degree of organization designed to implement the single-minded program of exterminating an entire group of people.[2] Thus, the Holocaust has become a paradigm for trauma. Is anyone safe? And when images of the embattled, wounded, starved, dispersed, and bereaved are broadcast on television, who remains untouched by trauma?

Psychologists and physicians have been aware of the impact of catastrophic events on personal stability at least since the beginning of the twentieth century—and even before when, in the middle of the nineteenth century, "reparations could be demanded from railway companies for suffering resulting from railway accidents."[3] Immediately after World War I, when the medical community recognized the existence of "shell shock" in front-line soldiers, Freud noted that "any excitations from outside which are powerful enough to break through the protective shield" can be described as traumatic and that such a "breach in an otherwise efficacious barrier against stimuli . . . provoke[s] a disturbance on a large scale in the [organism's] functioning."[4]

Freud understood that trauma, "an experience which . . . presents the mind with a stimulus too powerful to be dealt with, [inflicts] direct damage to . . . elements of the nervous system" and results in "permanent disturbances." He distinguished between sexually related psychological childhood injuries and "actual" neuroses. The latter, he postulated, could result "by chemical agency" from trauma sustained even in adulthood.[5] The research findings supporting Freud's position had to await sufficient progress in the development of scientific instrumentation and techniques, achieved in the 1990s.[6] Indeed, current investigations show that observable physical changes occur in the brain as a result of psychological trauma. Freud thought that actual neuroses could be cured more easily than the psychoneuroses. However, relieving adult-sustained trauma victims of their psychological symptoms has proved to be quite difficult, perhaps due to structural damage in the brain attendant to the traumatic experience. As one refugee from Nazi Germany put it, "You can't take it off with your clothes." She was right. Trauma penetrates the protective clothing, that is, "it gets under your skin"; and neither the purity of physical nor psychological nakedness is ever a protection against noxious excitation. The same has been noted in soldiers exposed to the physical devastation of war, loss of comrades, torture, brainwashing, fear, and other psychological suffering. It is clear that even in physically and psychologically sound individuals, a severe shock will manifest its "injurious effects,"[7] and trauma will be experienced when the individual surrenders to helplessness in the face of external (or internal) events, subjectively evaluated as vastly dangerous.[8]

Freud noted that preparedness and anxiety may "constitute the last line of defence of the shield against stimuli."[9] In fact, some findings show that previous experience with certain crises can provide an "inoculation perspective," thereby improving a person's ability to cope with future stresses.[10] According to an investigation of flood victims, elderly people who "had lived through a flood earlier in their lives endured a subsequent one with less anxiety." However, these findings have proved to be limited in application. Floods and other natural disasters are less pernicious in their psychological consequences than the calamities man inflicts upon man. Volcanoes, earthquakes, tornadoes, and floods leave death and destruction in their wake. In the face of such natural disasters man is often helpless and frightened. Yet given some warning, people can actively take precautions to protect themselves, their families, and their neighbors, and under certain circumstances, they can attempt to secure their property. If they survive, they may even have an opportunity to restore and rebuild. Then, having been through it once, victims are less vulnerable in later, similar situations. They can recognize the warning signals of disaster (and the concomitant anxiety) and have the knowledge required for making precautionary preparations and the skills to rebuild their lives. Having strengthened their physical and psychological defenses, they have reduced the risk of being traumatized.

Unfortunately, for combat soldiers and Holocaust survivors the evidence points in the direction of the "vulnerability perspective."[11] American World War II veterans with "high combat exposure" suffered greater posttraumatic stress disorder (PTSD) than other American veterans of the same war, even after an interval of forty years. A study of eighty World War II Dutch Resistance movement survivors found them to have more severe symptoms of PTSD eighteen to thirty-nine years later than they did immediately after the war. And a sample of men who had experienced both heavy combat and PTSD symptoms immediately after, suffered chronic physical ailments at the time of the research, decades later, or had died by age sixty-five.[12] Prisoners of war fared even worse: 67 percent of a sample of prisoners of war from the European and Pacific theaters of war were diagnosed with "lifetime" PTSD, though their symptoms were not correlated with any other mental disorders. Studies of Vietnam veterans also indicate "that both combat experience and exposure to atrocities hold negative life consequences."[13] Among Israeli soldiers, those exposed to the accumulated stress of multiple wars became more vulnerable and were less able to maintain their emotional equilibrium in battle. Zahava Solomon reasons that their increased vulnerability is due to the depletion of their "available coping resources" as a result of the multiple stresses and the "pathogenic effects of recurrent exposure" to war.[14] Hans Selye's seminal theories on stress and his animal experiments confirm the correctness of this view. Selye found that a reduction of (physical and psychic) resources follows repeated and accumulated stress.[15] He states that "adaptability is finite, exhaustion inexorably follows if the stressor is sufficiently severe and prolonged . . . and, if stress continues unabated, death ensues."[16]

It is hardly possible to compare the stresses of the World War II concentration-camp experience with those of the prisoners of war. These two groups were exposed to different sorts of physical torture and to different degrees of deprivation; the prisoners were at least somewhat shielded against starvation by the Geneva agreement.[17] Yet both these groups would seem to have been more impotent in their camp situations than a third group, the combat soldiers on the battlefield. As became clear over time, physical debilitation, as well as the deleterious psychological effects of impotence and passivity, are significant factors determining the intensity of the impact of a traumatic situation on its victims.

Psychological suffering was no small part of the trauma endured by a fourth group, the Holocaust victims who had not been incarcerated in concentration camps. Humiliations, prejudice, betrayal, and discrimination inflicted demoralizing psychic pain, long before knowledge of the killings in the extermination camps flooded them with horror, fear, loss, and mourning. Natural catastrophies can befall mankind indiscriminately. In war, the battles are fought between relative equals: Both maim and kill. But personal and social devaluation, torture, and the cruel extermination of one group of people by another also destroy fundamental human trust, so that victims of "human" disasters inflict greater "emotional damage than natural ones."[18]

It is, therefore, no surprise to learn that a subgroup of concentration-camp survivors (in a nonclinical sample of Holocaust survivors in Israel) were generally more pessimistic, more constricted in their thinking and in their personalities. Moreover, their general emotional health had been affected, as had the "emotional constellation of their children." On the other hand, concentration-camp survivors in Israeli reception camps were less pessimistic than other immigrants, and in accordance with the "inoculation perspective," could avail themselves of a variety of coping strategies. (One can speculate that for concentration-camp survivors, the Israeli reception camps were a great improvement and a relief, while other immigrants might have experienced extreme stress under the relatively primitive camp conditions in a climate to which they were absolutely unaccustomed.)

In Israel, the majority of Holocaust survivors did not manifest posttraumatic stress symptoms while they actively participated in building up the country, defending it, and rebuilding their lives.[19] Later, at an older age, passivity associated with reduced physical capacity and retirement left them vulnerable to an upsurge of previously suppressed (repressed) emotions.

Also, their legacy of helplessness vis-à-vis the Nazis intensified their reactions during the Gulf War, wherein Israel, when targeted by missiles, was pressured to refrain from retaliation. In contrast to those Israelis who had experienced fighting for themselves as a nation, the Holocaust survivors responded intensely to Hussein's "overwhelming malevolent power" and especially to his threat to make Israel into a "crematorium." Not only such a direct reference to the prior Holocaust trauma, but also events remotely reminiscent of previous trauma can trigger a reactivation of anxiety and other symptoms of an actual neurosis. "Trauma deepens trauma."[20]

Trauma is not limited to war, persecution, and natural disaster. It pervades societies all over the world. Today, despite some recent changes in accepted child-rearing patterns and in the status of women, physical and sexual abuse continues in all societies, inside as well as outside the home and family. Neighborhood shootings and burglaries have become daily events. Religious ideals, greed, and the thirst for power inspire vicious wars; the vengeance that follows fuels additional discrimination and torture. Violence is occurring in all cultures, in all ethnic and racial groups. And the victims are always vulnerable to traumatic stress. Though there may be some differences among the symptomatic manifestations, there is no doubt that posttraumatic stress disorders regularly occur in the victims, often in the witnesses, and, more frequently than we might suspect, in the perpetrators of violence.

The body of knowledge about the effects of trauma is growing rapidly. It is expanding by virtue of the technical innovations enabling research into brain function, and it is deepening in the sense that behavioral manifestations can now be understood more specifically in their relation to interactions between genetically determined temperament and environmental factors. While temperament, active or passive, sociable or shy, highly emotive or less so, remains a predictable thread throughout a person's life, it is as yet impossible to predict precisely the impact of particular events on an individual endowed with certain temperamental tendencies. Nevertheless, it is clear that traumatic experiences affect the brain pathways and that responses to traumatic events are colored by the relative flexibility or rigidity of a variety of mechanisms of defense. When these defensive barriers are shattered, the traumatic stimuli become more or less unmanageable, resulting in the nightmares, flashbacks, worries, fears, hostile outbursts, and depressive moods. The physiological changes observed in traumatized persons "are forever," and these persons remain vulnerable to repeated traumatization. They are "condemned to reexperience [parts of] the trauma" throughout their lives. And sometimes their subclinical symptoms may be as impeding as a full-blown posttraumatic stress disorder.[21]

The damaging effects of trauma are most severe in young children, both victims and perpetrators (or their offspring). Infant trauma "forms memory schemas" and can become an "organizer of [future] experience" or an "organizing principle."[22] The earlier the damage, the more crippling to the personality structure is its potential because the physical organisms of young children are delicate and their psychological development incomplete.[23] Their cognitive processes, defenses, and identifications are at risk of being distorted.[24] Some effects of the Nazi violence on two young boys, one Jewish and the other German, were brought to light during their respective analyses, begun in their early manhood in 1959.[25]

Together with his mother, the Jewish child, Jehuda, spent two years of his early childhood hiding from the Germans in a cave under a cow barn, without seeing the light of day. He was nearly blind by the time the Germans had been driven off. As a student years later, he lost his power of concentration and was tortured by anxieties, obsessions, and compulsions, as well as by fantasies of robots that he controlled. Various attempted cures resulted in a worsening of the condition until, close to psychosis, he consulted the psychotherapist, Anna Maria Jokl. The ensuing treatment revealed Jehuda's unconscious identification with vermin. Jokl points out that the Nazi murders, mutilations, tortures, and humiliations could becloud, but never extinguish, people's consciousness of being human. She believes that even in cases of brainwashing, the loss of identity is but temporary and the renunciation of ego and self-representation is a self-sacrifice for the sake of ending an unbearable loneliness, isolation, and ostracism. "But in this child, the unthinkable was achieved: because the Nazi ideology affected him prior to the development of his human identification, its formation was prevented and, *a priori*, in its stead was placed the self-representation of vermin." Unlike the brainwashed (who "confess" in order to be reinstated into a community and become once again "part of a whole"), as "vermin" Jehuda was unable to become a part of any unit inasmuch as "nowhere among the pictures in his unconscious could be found even a trace of an object (*die Spur eines Gegenüber*) to whom he could relate—not an accuser, not an enemy, no companion. He was alone: vermin." Even his mother's seemingly warm, protective relationship to him was deceptive in that she did not notice that he was "wounded unto death."[26]

Volker, the German, sought psychoanalytic treatment to relieve him of an almost unbearable tension: He suffered from attacks of jaundice and was ten pounds underweight. At home he kept an icy silence that, according to Jokl, was the camouflage of his internal chaos. His dreams and conscious fantasies revealed his hopelessness and the shattered state of the core of his being. As a young boy he had aspired to the Nazi ideals of toughness, pitilessness, and invulnerability. Yet it became evident in the SS (Nazi "storm trooper") boarding school that he was neither willing nor able to live up to these ideals. With searing shame he remembered nearly being beaten to death by a horde of strong, cruel classmates who saw him as weak and somewhat different. What a surprise it was, therefore, when, toward the end of his treatment, fierce hostility broke loose from his unconscious: insults, abuse, and violent national-socialist phrases shot out of his mouth, and before his eyes raging antisemitic pictures appeared, pictures of *Kristallnacht* (Night of Broken Glass) full of peculiar hate and fear of Jews—"Jews whom he had never known and emotions he could never have had" because at the time he was too young.[27] Volker recognized the "beast" in himself. He fantasized that the beast was isolated in a cave while life went on outside. Occasionally he fantasized that the beast ensnared a woman who would stroke him, then he killed her. He could not come out of the cave because, once seen, the beast would arouse fear, hate, and disgust. Volker discovered his "lust to torture, to treat human beings as garbage, and all that the Nazis had practiced to the bitter end."[28] Ultimately, the "beast" looked at his reflection in the mirror and there he saw "only unfathomable sadness."[29] At long last Volker could choose to confront the problem of his Nazi ancestors and seize the opportunity to unshackle himself from the chains of that evil legacy. But he was stuck with being a German, a link in a fatal chain. Unable to "cut himself off at the roots," he felt "sentenced to remain what I am. . . . I have no other fathers"—even if they left him poison as an inheritance. With the help of his therapist, Volker came to realize that Nazism was not the entirety of the German heritage. He learned to see himself as a link in another chain, too, that of German cultural accomplishments and traditions. Thus he was freed from having to cling to his poisoned roots and the toxic identifications of his youth, which later had made him so ill.

Anna Maria Jokl discovered the "horror of both sides . . . the son of the persecuted [and] the son of the persecutor." Both had been "damaged at their roots."[30] In this anthology, adults from many parts of the world have recorded their personal childhood horrors during and immediately after the Holocaust and World War II. The accounts of those events presented here and the efforts (in some cases belated) to master Holocaust-related experiences are paradigmatic for childhood social trauma and its aftermath. Some of the chapters in this volume help us understand how, as children and later in adulthood, survivors find sufficient energy and abilities to master their trauma. Supported by benign societal and familial conditions, survivors can surmount their injuries and, in most cases, fashion productive lives. This is borne out by some investigations of Holocaust survivors, including a number of the elderly. In about two-thirds of male survivors and one-third of female survivors, there is no evidence of "psychiatric impairments." Other studies reveal a higher level of anxiety, depression, and psychosomatic illness (especially gastrointestinal symptoms) than a control group. Despite this, survivors tend to have a significantly higher level of coping than a control group. They have "higher incomes, superior job histories, greater residential stability and lower divorce rates, [and are] more active in their communities, [showing] higher levels of altruism."[31]

Whatever the cause of stress and trauma, we now know that victims can be greatly helped by sympathetic, supportive listeners, whether these be friends or family, medical, or mental health practitioners. The deplorable fact is that for many years survivors of the Holocaust encountered too many people who were unprepared to listen. During several decades following World War II, even therapists often refrained from fully exploring the traumatic wartime experiences of their patients. Truly listening to those horrors puts the listener, including therapists, at risk of a "disruption in their schemas about self and the world." Therapists risk having their imagery and memory systems altered by the infiltration of the patients' traumatization, resulting in a "vicarious traumatization . . . [accompanied by] powerful affective states . . . [e.g.] sadness, anxiety, or anger." Who can give credence to the tales of violence, oppression, and abuse recounted by patients and still maintain a belief in a benign and meaningful world, a worthy self, and trustworthy people?[32]

We hope this volume will make a modest contribution toward a better understanding and toward amelioration of some of the pain of social trauma survivors—in all sectors of life and in all parts of the world—so that their trust, their ability to work, and their capacity to establish gratifying interpersonal relationships may be restored. The greatest benefit will accrue to their children when the generational transmission process of victimization is interrupted.

NOTES

1. William Clinton, Second Inaugural Address, "Transcript of President Clinton's Second Inaugural Address to the Nation," *New York Times*, January 21, 1997.

2. Daniel J. Goldhagen, *Hitler's Willing Executioners* (New York: Alfred A. Knopf, 1996).

3. Esther Fischer-Homberger, *Die traumatische Neurose: von somatischen zum sozialen Leiden* (Stuttgart und Wien: Verlag Hans Huber, 1975), 7.

4. Sigmund Freud, "Beyond the Pleasure Principle" (1920), in *The Standard Edition of the Complete Psychological Works of Sigmund Freud* (London: The Hogarth Press, 1955, 1964); 18:29 and "Introductory Lectures on Psychoanalysis: Fixation to Traumas—The Unconscious" (1915–1917) in *Standard Edition*, 16:275.

5. Freud, "Two Encyclopedia Articles" (1920), in *Standard Edition*, 18:243.

6. Ellen Gerrity and Susan Solomon, "The Treatment of PTSD and Related Stress Disorders: Current Research and Clinical Knowledge," in *Ethnocultural Aspects of Posttraumatic Stress Disorder*, ed. Anthony J. Marsella et al. (Washington, D.C.: American Psychological Association, 1996), 90, write, "Trauma is a psychobiological event . . . [with] potentially long-term neurobiological changes in the brain."

7. Sigmund Freud, "Analysis Terminable and Interminable" (1937), in *Standard Edition* (1964), 23:216–53, quote cited on 220.

8. Henry Krystal, "Trauma and Affects," in *The Psychoanalytic Study of the Child*, 53 vols. (New Haven, Conn.: Yale University Press, 1978), 33:95.

9. Freud, "Beyond the Pleasure Principle," 18:243.

10. Zahava Solomon, *Coping with War-Induced Stress* (New York: Plenum Press, 1995), 143.

11. Ibid.

12. Kimberly A. Lee, George Vaillant et al., "A Fifty Year Prospective Study of the Psychological Sequelae of World War II Combat," *American Journal of Psychiatry* 152 (1995): 516–22.

13. Elizabeth C. Clipp and Glen Elder, "The Aging Veteran of World War II: Psychiatric and Life Course Insights," in *Aging and Posttraumatic Stress Disorder*, ed. Paul E. Ruskin and John A. Talbott (Washington, D.C.: American Psychiatric Press, 1996).

14. Solomon, *Coping*, 143, 146.

15. Hans Selye, "The General Adaptation Syndrome and the Diseases of Adaptation," *Journal of Endocrinology* 6 (1946): 117–230; and idem, *The Physiology and Pathology of Exposure to Stress* (Montreal: Acta, 1950).

16. Hans Selye, "The Stress Concept Today," in *Handbook on Stress and Anxiety*, ed. Irwin L. Kutash et al. (San Francisco: Jossey-Bass, 1980), 129.

17. *Encyclopædia Britannica*, vol. 10 (1965): 100b. The original Geneva agreement of 1864 was revised in 1906 and extended to naval warfare at the second Hague peace conference in 1907.

18. Solomon, *Coping*, 151.

19. Shamai Davidson, personal communication, 1979.

20. Solomon, quoting Emanuel Berna in *Coping*, 154, 152.

21. Michael Hughes, M.D., "Psychic Trauma: Symptom Formation, Treatment, and Forensic Implications." Paper presented at the Symposium: Psychic Trauma—Clinical and Forensic Issues, American Psychological Association, 105th Annual Convention, August 15–19, 1997.

22. Karen Saakvitne, "Listening Beyond Words," *Contemporary Psychology* 41, no. 5 (1996): 505.

23. Gertrude Blanck and Rubin Blanck, *Ego Psychology: Theory and Practice* (New York: Columbia University Press, 1974).

24. J. C. Bringuier, *Conversations with Jean Piaget* (Chicago: Chicago University Press, 1980); Charlotte Kahn, "Cognitive Deficit and Management of the Closed Mind: Some Effects of Information Control after Fifty-seven Years of Totalitarianism in East Germany," *The Journal of Psychohistory* 19, no. 4 (Spring 1992): 409–20; Anna Freud, *The Ego and The Mechanisms of Defence* (1936; New York: International Universities Press, 1946).

25. Anna Maria Jokl, *"Zwei Fälle zum Thema 'Bewältigung der Vergangenheit'"* (Two cases on the subject of "coping with the past") (1965), *Leo Baeck Institut Bulletin, Jüdischer Verlag bei Athenäum* 8 (1988): 81–102.

26. Ibid., 84–85; trans. Charlotte Kahn.

27. Ibid., 95.

28. Ibid., 98.

29. Ibid., 96.

30. Ibid., 100.

31. Paul E. Ruskin and John A. Talbott, eds., "Conclusion," in *Aging and Posttraumatic Stress Disorder* (Washington, D.C.: American Psychiatric Press, 1996), 243–52.

32. Lisa McCann and Laurie Anne Pearlman, "Vicarious Traumatization: A Framework for Understanding the Psychological Effects of Working with Victims," *Journal of Traumatic Stress* 3, no. 1 (1991): 131–49.

Part I

PSYCHOHISTORICAL PERSPECTIVES

Charlotte Kahn

Time and time again, unbridled aggression has punctuated the history of man. Aggressive energy is a fact of life. It is also essential for the continuance of life, inasmuch as a measure of aggression is required for all accomplishments: from obtaining our livelihood to assuring our safety. However, extreme expressions of aggression pose a danger. Unrestrained aggression in the service of sadism, retaliation, and even aggression in the service of self-defense against perceived danger can create traumata for the objects of such aggression. It has always been so: Like dogs who snarl and attack when frightened, people viciously set upon people; and in each century ever more sophisticated weapons are invented to carry out personal and societally organized attacks. As the events of the twentieth century have shown, not only war among nations, but also the sadistic oppression of fellow citizens within their country can occur in even the most culturally advanced societies, leaving uncountable numbers of people to suffer both early and late onset of posttraumatic stress.

Humankind's inner resources of aggressive energy are inestimably difficult to harness. Though we may sugarcoat our hostile actions and soothe our feeble consciences with high ideals, we will stop at nothing to satisfy our wants and quell our anxieties. Though we struggle to tame our passionate desires and aim to act ethically, under the guise of a higher purpose we will destroy our fellow humans. These conflicts can play out within individuals, among their inner drives and prohibitions; between individuals and their clans, tribes, or societies; and among nations at war.

Whatever conditions, processes, and rationales seem to explain a historical event, fear and aggression seem to be paramount motivating factors. It seemed to Sigmund Freud that "idealistic motives served only as an excuse for the destructive appetites; and sometimes . . . idealistic motives . . .

pushed themselves forward in consciousness, while the destructive ones lent them an unconscious reinforcement."[1] In a 1932 letter to Freud, Albert Einstein stated, "man has within him a lust for hatred and destruction." This lust, he thought, could easily be raised to "the power of psychosis," and he wondered whether it is possible "to control man's mental evolution so as to make him proof against the psychoses of hate and destructiveness."[2] What began as "domination by brute violence" developed into "violence supported by intellect." And as the power of a community exceeds the strength of individuals, "we see that right is the might of a community. It is still violence . . . [and] works by the same methods and follows the same purposes."[3]

Freud's formula for indirectly "combat[ing]" war is to bring "Eros, its antagonist, into play against it" either by loving relations or by identification with others, because "the structure of human society is . . . based on" identifications.[4] Human societies attempt to regulate aggression by taboos, mores, and principles that are imparted by the society's representatives to each generation of children. First in the home, parents (perhaps also older siblings or other relatives) offer themselves as models of identification and socialize young children. Ideally, this occurs in an atmosphere of comfort and trust, engendering optimism and self-confidence, until children are ready to venture out into the community. Then teachers, mentors, and law-enforcement officers continue the task of shaping members of the community and inducting them into the society. The goal is to preserve the regulated social functions and to protect the fundamental trust required for social cohesion on all levels: individual, familial, and societal. Under benign conditions, the socialization process results in sublimation; thus, in a modulated form, aggressive energy continues to be available for achieving constructive personal and societal goals. As "assertiveness," aggression becomes a highly valued personality trait, particularly in Western societies.

Undisciplined persons, on the other hand, can cause great harm to themselves, to their victims, and to their society at large. When an unmodulated aggression fuels the survival instinct, it may be expressed as an impulsive physical attack, unrestrained greed, or vicious verbal abuse. These behaviors inflict pain, loss, and denigration, and disrupt the social fabric. Especially when people feel endangered and frightened, hatred toward the threatening object may infuse their aggressive drive, turning it into sadism.[5] Inflicting hurt on an enemy—real or imagined—releases the tension created by fear. And the pleasure of the relief, in turn, can reinforce the sadistic behavior until it becomes a habitual response.[6] In some persons, the shame (rather than remorse) accompanying sadistic behavior arouses additional anger in its wake, complicating and perpetuating the further-inflamed sadism. This, in turn, leads to further traumatization and victimization of the object of the aggression.

As hurtful and destructive as this process is in individual and family relations, aggression is magnified when socially sanctioned and institutionalized. Moreover, modern technology has made possible the implementation of both the personal sadistic drives and the societal destructive aggression— with catastrophic results. No less than individuals, communities direct hostile aggression against real or perceived threats to physical survival (economic and/or territorial), and against intruders threatening to dilute or annihilate the existing civilization by importing their own, different culture. That is how the Nazi regime saw the Jewish citizens of Germany, and this perceived threat to the "pure" German culture and people became the guiding motivation to persecute and exterminate the Jews—leaving survivors as well as many of their progeny traumatized. However, even in a country of immigrants such as the United States, newcomers to the society are greeted with an intense ambivalence: They are welcomed as instruments of renewal, feared as economic competitors, and reviled as destroyers of the dominant character of the country.[7] Fortunately, in the United States, behavioral expression of these xenophobic attitudes is not sanctioned by law.

Xenophobia also exists in the animal world. Depending upon their social organization—into unconnected individuals, families, or colonies (e.g., of birds), or into tribes (e.g., of rats)—aggression may be focused on the defense of a territory or, according to Konrad Lorenz, against "every member of the species that belongs to a different tribe." And, he continues, "in order to channel aggression along harmless paths," evolution has " 'invented' " some useful mechanisms such as rituals, and in man, "responsible morality" is of great importance.[8]

Despite the very many explorations by philosophers, historians, and psychologists, a complete understanding of the pervasive individual and cultural animosity to difference still eludes us. Perhaps this phenomenon can be illuminated from three perspectives: individual development, biological evolution, and sociocultural continuity. Attempting to account for the prevalence of xenophobia on the individual level, one cannot ignore infants' "stranger anxiety" as a possible precursor. Stranger anxiety is experienced by infants when they become aware of the difference between mother and an unfamiliar person. Expecting the comfort and familiarity of mother's face and embrace, they may be overwhelmed with disappointment and fear when confronted by a stranger. Viewed biologically, specifically genetically, the degree of protection offered another individual is in direct proportion to a shared gene pool and is motivated by the biological imperative to hold one's "immortal genes in trust for the future."[9] Sociologically stated, the individual instinct for self-preservation is extended to the kinship group, the tribe, or a *Volk*. Transposed to a cultural point of view, it would mean that members of a society are intent on preserving their civilization by means of a multigenerational transmission process of education, imitation, and identification. A "unit of cultural transmission" has been posited as a possible equivalent of the biological replicator (the gene) and labeled *meme*.[10]

The concept of meme might be of help in understanding the current tribal and national belligerencies in the Balkans, in Southeast Asia, and in Africa. The traumatization of the enemy's women and children attendant to wars points to the possibility that the "selfish gene"[11] and the conservative meme are influencing the sociobiological process and fueling the deadly conflicts, as manifested in the sadistic behaviors and their aftermath. To wit, Hutus in Africa committed genocide, killing 500,000 Tutsi men, and while "rape in Rwanda was uncommon . . . during the genocide, women became deliberate targets" of rape for the Hutus, who assaulted 250,000 Tutsi women. In light of the theory of the "selfish gene" and meme, it is not totally surprising that the Hutus raped; nor is it surprising that once violated by enemy males (especially after having borne the enemy's children) the Tutsi women are now ostracized by their own people, their "personal and community integrity" destroyed. These circumstances, worsened by wretched poverty, gives meaning to some Tutsi women's practice of infanticide—a desperate extension of the killing. In their closed society, Tutsi women are reluctant to express their suffering openly, but health workers have observed their trauma symptoms: nightmares, sleep disorders, psychosomatic ills, withdrawal, and general dysfunction. Surviving Tutsi children, already traumatized by what they have witnessed and by having been orphaned, continue to face mortal danger. To save their lives, relatives hide them in the bush at night.[12]

The sociobiological perspective might also add to our understanding of antisemitism. For most of their history, Jews have lived in the Diaspora, where their "different" culture often has been experienced as a threat. Jews have been "strangers" beginning with their stay in Egypt during biblical times. As told in the story of Exodus, both the Egyptians and the Israelites (the ancestors of the Jews) struggled to preserve their own memes. Throughout their history (as will be described in chapter 1), Jews have to a great extent protected their gene pool and preserved their civilization against external influences by injunctions against intermarriage, especially when the social boundaries between themselves and others became threateningly permeable.

How these dynamics have played themselves out in the lives of Holocaust victims will be discussed from a psychohistorical perspective in the first section of this book. In the first chapter, "The Background of Persecution and Its Aftermath," Milton Jucovy provides a historical perspective on apocalypse, xenophobia, internecine struggles, antisemitism, and the choice of Jews as targets of fury. Jucovy shows that a demoralized, humiliated, yet physically vigorous German population was inspired by a charismatic leader—the people's messianic deliverer—to rid German society of "pathogenic organisms," the impediments to the realization of that nation's destiny. The Nazis believed Germany had to be cleansed of the "defilers"—the Jews, as well as Gypsies, homosexuals, and the mental or physically impaired—to remain a "pure" German nation and culture. Jucovy goes on to show that the surviving victims of such a purging process may be seriously affected, as exposure to external trauma coalesces with an existing unconscious anxiety to create psychic conflict. Some survivors of the Nazi persecution speak freely about their experiences, while others remain silent. During a postulated "latency period" after World War II, the subject of the Holocaust was frequently avoided, even by psychoanalysts and the survivors undergoing psychological treatment. On the part of the German officials in charge of allocating indemnification to Nazi victims, there was a great reluctance to recognize the late-appearing symptoms of the Holocaust trauma.[13] A case example is put forward here and the possibility of pretraumatic pathology discussed.

In his chapter, "Historical Trauma: Psychohistorical Reflections on the Holocaust," Robert Prince writes about the Holocaust and its implication for future threats of mass destruction of a magnitude heretofore unknown, but made possible by technological advances. He draws attention to a new category of evil-doers, the "desk-killers." Prince finds a connection between the disruption of faith in the social order, caused by the enormity of Holocaust evil, and a search for order. This search may be manifested in the victims' attempts at mastery by repetitively re-experiencing the trauma. Prince debunks three "myths" about Holocaust victims: the regressed behavior of concentration-camp prisoners—belied by a frequently observed ability to maintain interpersonal relations and personal dignity; the reluctance of survivors to speak—refuted by a "felt obligation to the dead to speak," though often the listeners did not want to hear; and the presumed "survivor syndrome" and "survivor guilt"—reframed as an attempt to maintain "ties with lost objects."

Judith S. Kestenberg writes about "Adult Survivors, Child Survivors, and Children of Survivors." She defines "adult survivors" as those who lived through the Holocaust as grown-ups and "child survivors" who survived the Holocaust as children with their parents or alone. As a group, child survivors mourn their lost childhood, yet tend to "self-heal" by striving to become quite indistinguishable from other, nonpersecuted children in their surroundings. "Children of survivors" are defined as those born after World War II. While their parents may be self-deprecating, feeling depressed and defeated, or may overachieve to compensate, their children are often delegated to restore the parents' losses. The numerous ways of performing this impossible task, and the concurrent conflicts, are the main focus of this chapter.

Kazimierz Godorowski explains in "Man Behind Walls" that previously adaptive behaviors and values became inappropriate in the inhumane settings of the ghetto and the concentration camp. The psychological and physical effects of life under ghetto and camp conditions are described, with special attention given to observable personality changes. Many of these changes can be ascribed to the inadequacy of "supplies" to maintain a physiological balance. The permanent condition of hunger rendered the inmates "vulnerable to any manipulation" and some were tempted to collaborate with their oppressors in order to obtain food. Three phases of change are postulated: preoccupation with food, loosening of moral restraints, and apathy.

In chapter 5, "Interviewing for Indemnification," Milton Kestenberg recounts some of his experiences as an attorney representing Holocaust survivors. The West German indemnification laws—intended to compensate victims for their material, psychological, and physical suffering at the hands of the Nazis—were administered extremely unsympathetically and were undermined by the rigidity within the German medical and judicial systems. Intimidated Holocaust victims often were unable to prove past experiences as the root of their present physical and emotional disorders because, under the pressure of the examinations, they did not recall certain events or failed to link memories of past events with current ailments. Case examples illustrate this lawyer's sensitive, therapeutic interview methods designed to elicit and connect pieces of information that were then woven into an acceptable application for indemnification.

"Impact on the Second and Third Generations," by Eva Fogelman, indicates that the children of Holocaust survivors are generally not more psychologically impaired than their peers. However, when pathology does occur, its onset is often connected to "anniversary reactions," reaching the age of their parents' traumatization, or to Holocaust-related events, such as exposure to dangerous situations. Sometimes, bearing a resemblance to a deceased member of the family or having been given that person's name may interfere with these children's formation of their own distinctive identities. Some children of survivors may have difficulties synthesizing their image of the deceased ancestor whose name they carry with their experience of their own unique attributes, causing them to feel inauthentic. Any healing process must give consideration to the conflicts, defenses, and unconscious mechanisms relating to one's name before identity integration can take place.

"Antisemitism and Jewish Identity in Hungary Between 1989 and 1994," by Judit Mészáros, is a comparative study of sociopolitical trends relating to antisemitism under the former communist regime in Hungary and now in the young democracy. In different ways, each epoch had an impact on Jewish identity. The chapter is based on sociological studies, interviews, and clinical experiences with first and second generation Holocaust survivors.

NOTES

1. Sigmund Freud, "Why War?" (1932), in *The Standard Edition of the Complete Psychological Works of Sigmund Freud* (London: The Hogarth Press, 1964), 22:197–215, quote cited on 210.

2. Albert Einstein, quoted in Freud, "Why War," 201.

3. Freud, "Why War?" 205.

4. Ibid., 212.

5. The combination of hostile aggression and sexuality also results in sadism.

6. David P. Barash, *Sociobiology and Behavior* (New York: Elsevier, 1977), 221–22.

7. Paul Elovits and Charlotte Kahn, eds., *Immigrant Experiences: Personal Narrative and Psychological Analysis* (Madison and Teaneck, N.J.: Fairleigh Dickinson University Press, 1997), 11–12.

8. Konrad Lorenz, *On Aggression* (New York: Harcourt Brace & World, 1966), xii.

9. Richard Dawkins, *The Selfish Gene* (New York: Oxford University Press, 1976), 71.

10. Ibid., 206. He explains that "meme" is an abbreviation of the Greek word "*mimime*" and can be related to "memory" or the French word "*meme*," meaning "same."

11. Ibid.

12. Elizabeth Royte, "The Outcasts," *New York Times Magazine*, January 19, 1997, 37–39.

13. William Niederland, *Folgen der Verfolgung: das Überlebenden Syndrom in Seelenmord* (Consequences of persecution: Survivng the syndrome of soul-murder) (Frankfurt am Main: Suhrkamp, 1968).

1

The Background of Persecution and Its Aftermath

Milton Jucovy

INTRODUCTION

The twentieth century will shortly make its exit, leaving a legacy of blood-baths far in excess of any equivalent historical time frame. Among the most infamous are the massacre of Armenians by the Turks, the atomic attacks on Hiroshima and Nagasaki by the U.S. Air Force, the dispersion and "killing fields" devised by the Khmer Rouge and the Pol Pot government in Cambodia, and the recent devastation and civil wars in the former Yugoslavia and in various African countries. The massive destruction wrought by the Nazi regime during the Holocaust, in which a sophisticated technology was applied to the relentless and highly organized slaughter of an entire people and the extermination of millions in German-occupied territories, stands out as a paradigm of persecution. The Final Solution, a concept adopted by the Nazi regime to plan, implement, and then fulfill an ideology of hate, was an apocalyptic end in itself.

Attempts to comprehend fully the dark forces unleashed during the Holocaust have met only limited success. Many Holocaust survivors have warned us that we can never understand their experiences completely. Elie Wiesel has asked, "How do you tell children—big and small—that society could lose its mind and start murdering its own soul? How do you unveil horrors without offering at the same time some measure of hope?"[1] Undertaking a scientific study of this period of infamy poses an almost insuperable challenge. It may even be presumptuous to attempt rationally, soberly, and as objectively as possible to speak of the unspeakable and to describe the indescribable. Yet, some understanding may be achieved by applying the prism of psychoanalysis to living memories.

The term "Holocaust" presents a semantic problem. It has been criticized as having a euphemistic ring and obscuring the general concept of genocide, thus diminishing the Jewish victims of Nazi tyranny. However, it is precisely this term the Jewish people themselves have chosen in the English language to describe their fate of persecution and death.[2] The term used in Hebrew is *shoah*. While the word "Holocaust" denotes great destruction and devastation, its etymological roots suggest a more specific, Jewish interpretation. It is derived from the Greek word *holokauston*, a translation in the *Septuagint* (Greek version of the Old Testament) for the Hebrew word *olah*, which means "what is brought up." Translated into English, *olah* can mean "an offering made by fire unto the Lord," or a burnt offering, implying that once more the Jewish people are sacrificial victims and that the Holocaust is another link in the chain of Jewish suffering and martyrdom.[3]

While the Jewish historical experience of recurrent persecution has claimed many lives and caused untold suffering, the catastrophe of the Holocaust—involving the death of 6 million and the agony of many others— was slaughter on a scale surpassing violent antisemitic crimes of the past and it transcended all previous ordeals. It consumed the majority of Eastern European Jews and destroyed an entire civilization.

ANTISEMITISM

In general, past explorations of antisemitism have been more useful in describing its phenomenology and applications than in understanding its deep-rooted causes. A joining of forces by psychoanalysts and historians, based on their common absorption with the past and a shared interest in problems of causality, might deepen future investigations of antisemitism. This natural partnership has not been forged altogether fruitfully as yet, but remains a hoped-for goal.[4]

Hardly an optimist, Freud nevertheless expressed the hope that the process of civilization and an evolution of culture might enable the human race to govern its instinctual life and help to sublimate aggressive impulses.[5] Freud was writing during a period of apparent enlightenment and emancipation that ended in ashes and skeletons, and in the disappearance of a rich and lively European Jewish culture. Psychoanalysts whose study is anchored in clinical material have had some success in linking antisemitism to developmental issues, such as "stranger anxiety" in infants and xenophobia in adults. It is also important to differentiate more clearly among the varieties of antisemitic expression, as these cannot always be regarded as pathological phenomena, especially when embedded in a cultural matrix regarding antisemitism as normal and acceptable within certain boundaries defined by the community. Therefore, we should distinguish prejudice from a more virulent form of antisemitism, which, in its ultimate expression, may explode in activities that can lead to genocide. Fortunately, in most instances the relatively mild expression of antisemitic prejudice remains on the same level of lack of taste and sensitivity as other xenophobic attitudes.

Xenophobia is also manifest in various segments of the Jewish community in the form of prejudices related to places of birth, degree of assimilation, or to religious affiliation. Indeed, throughout recorded history, members of the same religious and ethnic groups have on occasion reviled or even attacked one another, and the same phenomenon has appeared among Jews.

From Paganism to the Consolidation of Antisemitism

Although internecine prejudice was rampant in the pagan polytheistic world and a zealous antipaganism prevailed, prior to the sixth century B.C.E. pre-Christian antisemitism was not particularly apparent.[6] The practical polytheism and political tolerance of the Greco-Roman world did not easily lend itself to a fanatical hatred of the Jewish community, although outbursts against the Jews in Alexandria punctuated this period. The events seemed to have been fueled by the refusal of the Jewish community to join other citizens in a communal sacrifice. The dietary laws of the Jews and the Jewish prohibition of intermarriage contributed to these eruptions of antisemitic feeling.

Antisemitism appeared in Roman society after the destruction of the temple, as documented by the Roman historian, Tacitus, who accused Jews of, among other things, not sacrificing their children. However, the crucial event establishing Western antisemitism was the ultimate triumph of Christianity over the Roman Empire. At first, the Roman world and the early church thought of Christianity as but another monotheistic, antipagan, and exclusively Jewish sect. Ironically, Jewish Christians later introduced an intensified degree of antisemitism. This was related to the Gospels of St. John and the Evangelists, who developed the doctrine that God had renounced His covenant with the Jews and established one with the followers of Jesus. Paul, after experiencing his epiphany, rejected the early Christian belief that a convert must first become Jewish to "know" Christ, and with his followers, promulgated the doctrine that God had indeed abandoned the Jews, substituting the gentiles as His chosen people. This crucial exclusion more easily allowed the Jews to become the target of aggression in myth and in deed.

When the Germanic tribes were converted to Christianity as a result of Paul's apostolic efforts, they had little difficulty in accepting the hostility of the early church fathers.[7] By modern standards, these early clerical writings contained some of the most bizarre descriptions of Jews imaginable, suggesting a multitude of anatomical features with Satanic and hermaphroditic qualities. Prevailing opinion suggests that significant antisemitism was visited on the Jewish people when St. Paul established the church as a gentile institution and assigned guilt in the death of Jesus to Jewish leaders and priests.[8]

Although the more virulent forms of antisemitism waned to some extent in the twentieth century, they still arose sporadically, not least in the Mendel Beilis case and in the passionate promotion by Henry Ford of *The Protocols of the Elders of Zion*.[9] The blood libel was at least partly replaced by myths about money and race. Among antisemites, Jews were now regarded in polarized fashion as materialistic and devoid of religious ideals and values. They were regarded as both reclusive and pushy, frugal and ostentatious, cold and hypocritically oversentimental. It becomes evident, then, that the search for meaning and causality of the dark, malignant events of the Holocaust cannot be found solely in clinical observations of individual xenophobia.[10] To explain the progression of antisemitism from sentiment to significant political movement, it is necessary to look beyond the individual and to examine society itself. For example, the combination of a crisis-like sociopolitical environment and an atmosphere of general despair may engender feelings of violence, resulting in a need to find scapegoats. In addition, prevalent "myths" (such as a generally accepted belief that Jews are Christ-killers), plus a leader who senses and expresses the general despair and also seems to point to a way out of the crisis (despite the fact that he may be very disturbed), contribute to an antisemitic movement of dangerous proportions.

THE RISE OF NAZI POWER

Before he took power, when German bishops questioned Hitler about his anti-Jewish policies, he answered that he was only institutionalizing what had been preached and practiced in Germany for nearly two centuries.[11] Expressions of antisemitism had held sway from the early centuries of the Common Era until the premonitory rumblings of the Holocaust began after the collapse of the Weimar Republic, at which time the National Socialist Party came to power in Germany under Hitler and his henchmen. The Nazis socialized the fluctuating, more or less latent, genocidal and sociopathic inclinations in the masses, inciting them to war and to the elimination of a racially "impure" people.[12] This served to block the awareness of despair, self-hatred, and crushing feelings of inferiority among the German population. This formulation resonates with the thesis that Nazi physicians working in the concentration camps were able to see mass murder as a healing and cleansing process. In a desperate striving for new life and vitality, they linked mass murder to the medical metaphor of healing by extirpating any pathogenic organisms infecting a body or, in this case, the society.[13] The majority of the population was placed in a trancelike state, the awareness of their humanity lost. As military defeat in World War II loomed, Germany inexorably became a death factory, demonstrating the dangers inherent in a collective search for symbols of power. The people who felt impotent and were consumed by rage overwhelmed a society otherwise wearing a most civilized facade. It was a very bitter irony that Germany, once a paradigm for assimilation, meted out torture and death to its Jewish community.

APOCALYPTIC PHENOMENA AND THE HOLOCAUST

When prejudices are examined in individual treatment, certain patterns may emerge, as well as a broad range of conflicts, their points of origin, and modes of conflict resolution.[14] It would be helpful similarly to understand how groups can become involved in a broad social movement that persecutes a component societal group. The dominant group then behaves as though subject to an imperative that takes priority over any observable individual differences. This is the case in apocalyptic movements, many of which have had an important bearing on the vicissitudes of violent forms of antisemitism.

Militant apocalyptics treasure the illusion of rebirth into a messianic age, an illusion reflecting their destructive and reconstructive proclivities. These apocalyptic fantasies may be compared to the delusions of a passive schizophrenic who, often chronically catatonic, decathects the world of reality and fashions delusions about its rebirth. The more violently inclined schizophrenic has militant fantasies, impelling him first to destroy everyone around him and then himself. The violent schizophrenic identifies with a violent leader, one such as Hitler. In a reconstructive mood, the same person will identify with a more benign messianic savior.[15] Presumably, the goal is to eradicate what must be unbearable pain.

An apocalyptic vision appeared in the Jewish community during the Hasmonean period (close to the beginning of the second century B.C.E.) when it was "revealed" that at the "end of days," enemies and persecutors of the local population would be eradicated by the good angels of God, who would then save the righteous remnant of Israel. This mystical enlightenment replaced an intolerable reality by offering a sense of a hospitable universe and a caring presence who will ultimately punish the enemy and reward the believer.[16]

The promise of a rebirth of the righteous furnishes comfort to those powerless to alleviate their misery and encourages a passive messianic tradition. Problems arise when programs for activism become acceptable and encourage the impatient and reckless to form armies to fight on the side of the good angels of God against their demonic antagonists.

Although the official Christian church tended to discourage apocalyptic thinking, fantasy gave way to activism in the fifth century of the Common Era and foreshadowed the Crusades that enveloped Europe during the Middle Ages. During the height of the Black Death in the middle of the fourteenth century, waves of apocalyptics, the Flagellants, fell upon the Jews, whom they blamed for poisoning the wells. The Flagellants claimed their actions were designed to please God, although they were violating official church doctrine, which held that Jews were also perishing from the plague. Rootless and desperate indigents from northern France and western Germany, demoralized by famine, floods, and illness, also joined the First and Second Crusades. They were incited by leaders whose fanaticism convinced them that the deliverance of Jerusalem required nothing less than the destruction of Islam in the Holy Land and of the Jews at home.[17]

The selection of Jews as targets of Crusader fury has been explained variously by religious tradition, social mythology, and economic rivalry. One intriguing suggestion is that, in the face of inner or outer stress, anti-Jewish hostility may serve to draw defensive boundaries to deter the frequent crossing of group boundaries occurring in times of comfort and prosperity. Society may withdraw from xenophilia and exogamy during crises, and, with the aid of mythology, may draw the boundaries closer. This hypothesis might account for the fluctuations in a community's responses to Jews.

Moreover, the mechanism may be reciprocal, inasmuch as boundaries are also used by the Jewish community to insure its survival. Thus, in an unusually benign and accepting environment, the Jewish community may perceive the situation as an appealing and seductive invitation to exogamous marriages, and ultimately as a threat of assimilation, loss of identity, and extinction. Reactive retrenchment may well include a traditional response that asserts a more vigorous retreat to separateness, or *havdallah* as it is known in Hebrew. Often perceived as a xenophobic attitude by the non-Jewish community, this defensive position can play into the very hands of those who would demonize Jews. In this way, Jews may then suffer varying degrees of persecution instead of extinction through assimilation.[18]

In short, apocalyptic movements tend to appear in a demoralized, humiliated, but still physically vigorous, population.[19] They are inspired by a charismatic leader who is seen as a messianic deliverer. Both the populace and its leader harbor unacknowledged self-contempt and impulses toward self-destruction, feelings that are projected onto a scapegoat. While optimism and hope can, for a time, create the illusion that there will be a rebirth into a messianic age of marvelous tranquility, self-destructive features are revealed by the ultimate failure of many such movements, as the leaders and their followers meet defeat and perish in death.

Examination reveals how closely the Nazi phenomenon resembles the pattern of apocalyptic thinking. Hitler's apocalyptic vision facilitated projection of evil onto the Jews, to whom he attributed Satanical power. The self-destructive aspect surfaced when Hitler declared that if the German people were unwilling to sacrifice everything for their self-preservation, they deserved to disappear—and he was barely deterred from carrying out their destruction, along with his own.

THE NEED TO FORGET

In 1945 the war in Europe was over, and the advancing Allied forces liberated the concentration and death camps, shocked by what they encountered. The survivors tried to find a place among the living once again, some attempted to take up life in the towns and countries from which they had been deported. There they found desolation and, in many places, encountered hostility manifest to the point of outright death threats. While awaiting their visas to immigrate to more receptive and congenial places abroad, large numbers of the impoverished and stateless survivors were cared for temporarily in displaced persons camps. Many survivors who tried to make their way to Palestine before 1948 were intercepted by the British and sent to internment camps in Cyprus. Those who succeeded in reaching the shores of the "Promised Land" soon had to confront the ordeals of the Israeli War of Independence, followed by the evacuation of British forces and the creation of the Jewish state. A fairly sizable number of survivors were able to make contact with family members in the United States, Canada, Argentina, and other countries in South America, and to obtain visas allowing them to settle in these countries.

During the first years after their liberation, the energies of the survivors were absorbed by finding a way back to some semblance of conventional life. Most had to learn a new language, search for other occupations, and meet the challenges of the society and culture of a foreign land. Many families clung together, hoping to recreate their original communities in new neighborhoods, but in effect creating new ghettos. They were surrounded by an alien culture that, though not usually physically threatening, nevertheless regarded the newcomers with a degree of awe and mistrust, thereby presenting the very embodiment of a past the survivors wanted to forget. It was rare for a family to have survived intact. New partners found each other among fellow survivors and started new families. Life was safer and more bearable, but adaptation was by no means easy.

The shock and drama of liberation and the need to address the physical plight of the victims of Nazi persecution helped mobilize active assistance and held survivors before the eyes and, for a time, in the conscience of the world. Then, for at least two powerful reasons, a curtain of silence descended. First, although the Jewish people can be seen as a group united by common trauma, for close to a decade following World War II intense individual and collective defense mechanisms warded off the preoccupation with their painful recent history and the memories of traumatic experiences.[20]

Despite the long history of exiles and pogroms, almost nothing in that history prepared the Jewish community for Hitler's Final Solution. Statements such as "Nobody told us" or "We couldn't imagine or believe what we saw" are found frequently in archival Holocaust documents. During the decade after 1945, survivors had a compelling need to deny and repress their experiences. The Hebrew writer Aharon Appelfeld, who arrived in Israel after his liberation from a concentration camp at the age of twelve, gave the following retrospective account: "After liberation the one desire was to sleep, to forget, and to be reborn. At first, there was a wish to talk incessantly about one's experiences; this gave way to silence, but learning to be silent was not easy. When the past was no longer talked about, it became unreal, a figment of one's imagination. The new Israeli identity, sun-burned, practical, and strong, was grafted upon the old identity of the helpless victim. Only in nightmares was the past alive, but then even dreaming ceased."[21]

What appeared to be a moderately healthy and adaptive way of dealing with the Holocaust could be achieved only with massive denial and repression of the traumatic period. It is not surprising, therefore, that the intolerable memories of the past eventually returned to haunt the survivor. And so it was for a woman who, as a child, had been removed from the Warsaw ghetto and raised secretly by a Catholic family. Both her parents had been killed, and she was later found by an aunt. She said, "For years I claimed in a big way that I did not suffer from the war, that I was a privileged child in the ghetto. I was lucky to have been much loved by my mother and aunt who raised me. Then this whole defensive edifice gave way little by little," and after some time she realized that "the much-loved child really suffered a succession of abandonments." The aunt who had rescued her from the ghetto abandoned her when she was ten, by leaving for Israel. In retrospect she thinks, "It was just revenge for [my having] survived her daughter and her sister." The privilege of survival weighs heavily on her. She admits that, "Life seems very hard to me and I live it from day to day without projects as if I could only hold my head above water and [were] incapable of doing the least bit for others."[22]

The second reason for silence was a counterpart to the survivors' need to forget: The world needed to forget. One concentration-camp survivor reported that he "regularly made the observation that people did not really want me to talk about my experiences and whenever I started, they invariably showed their resistance by interrupting me, by asking me to tell them how I got out."[23] And Elie Wiesel wrote,

Had we started to speak, we would have found it impossible to stop. Having shed one tear, we would have drowned the human heart. So invincible in the face of death and the enemy, we now felt helpless. We were met with disbelief. People refused to listen, to understand, to share. There was a division between us and them, between those who endured and those who read about it, or would refuse to read about it. We thought people would remember our experiences, our testimony, and manage to suppress their violent impulses to kill or to hate.[24]

PERIOD OF NEGLECT

Early plans to rehabilitate the traumatized population emphasized material assistance while psychological issues were ignored. Psychiatrists and psychoanalysts neglected to confront the psychological problems of survivors. One notable exception to this extraordinary oversight was provided by Paul Friedman, who surveyed the mental health of Jewish displaced persons in Europe and paid special attention to the problems of children.[25] Under the auspices of the American Joint Distribution Committee, he also helped establish a program of mental hygiene for Palestine. Friedman's work was thus one of the earliest efforts to focus attention on the vast extent of psychic trauma, which was later to be exhaustively investigated and described.

During this period of "latency," when silence, denial, avoidance, and repression reigned, psychotherapists were hampered by their own reluctance to face the facts of the Holocaust.[26] Enormous temporal and emotional distances needed to be traversed before defenses mobilized to deal with the tragedies of the past could be abandoned—before survivors were able to cope with their repressed memories and before well-trained and experienced mental health professionals were ready to deal with issues crying out for confrontation and intervention.

The legislation passed by the Federal German Republic in the early 1950s, providing indemnification to victims of Nazi persecutions, helped to bridge the gap, though at first only physical infirmities were considered for indemnification. Only since 1965 have psychiatric conditions been recognized as possible results of persecution. According to traditional German medical theories, any traumatic experience affecting the psychic apparatus, no matter how severe, could have only temporary aftereffects on the individual. Arbitrarily, late-appearing sequelae of trauma and more permanent disorders were considered genetic and thus unrelated to persecution. Furthermore, the German psychiatrists contended that since individuals who spent their first two or three years of life in a concentration camp or in hiding will not be able to recall the details of that suffering, these traumata cannot be psychologically damaging. This opinion is certainly not supported by modern findings.

In an exceptional case, one patient was declared disabled and a pension awarded. In 1944, as a five-year-old boy, this man had been deported from Hungary with his parents and then assigned to a group subjected to mass shooting. He lay among the corpses for days, until he was rescued by local people and hidden until liberation. After the war, he regularly hid under tables and benches and was afraid of all adults, a disturbance that later developed into delusions about imaginary agents. He was hospitalized with the diagnosis of a paranoid illness and was granted an indemnification on the premise that while schizophrenia cannot be created by persecution alone, a psychotic episode may be precipitated by a traumatic experience.[27] During the ensuing few years, this decision proved to be an exception, as the role of persecution in determining emotional disturbance continued to be overlooked.[28]

Experiences with clients, however, were convincing—often more so than psychiatric reports. For example, the claim of a young suicidal woman suffering from learning disabilities, fear of using public transportation, stranger anxiety, and depression was rejected on the basis of absence of a causal relationship between her current condition and her earlier experiences— even though she had been born in a concentration camp where her father had died. Ultimately, her claim was sustained in the form of a lump-sum settlement.[29]

Another poignant example is Moshe: At age seven he suffered a forced separation from his father, who was taken to a labor camp; the murder of his mother by the Nazis shortly thereafter; his own deportation to a concentration camp; and the witnessing of his twin brother's extermination.

After liberation, Moshe graduated from a "rabbinical school" in a displaced persons' camp and was then employed as a clerk in a small company. Brought there by a co-worker every morning and directed to his tasks, he functioned like an automaton until the end of the workday, when his co-worker would bring him home again. Once home with his wife and two children, he remained mute throughout the evening meal and stared at the ceiling thereafter, until retiring for the night. In his sleep, however, he would find his voice—screaming as a result of terrifying nightmares.

During the meeting with his attorney, Moshe did not utter one word. His wife did the talking and said that he always acted this way. She claimed she had children with him only because he had raped her and indicated she could not take this life any longer.

Moshe's application for reparations was rejected on the grounds that his seemed to be a classical instance of a childhood experience, which does not necessarily leave a traumatic mark on an individual. Seemingly, this arbitrary decision was made on insufficient evidence and was reversed when it was learned that while attending the rabbinical school, Moshe had clung to a particular teacher, speaking to no one else and never playing with other children. Ironically, most of this information had been available to the original examiner, who had disregarded it as irrelevant.[30]

Despite the complications and controversies inherent in implementing the restitution legislation, the laws were well intentioned and helped bring the survivors' plight to the attention of the world once more. There was also a redramatization of the harrowing concentration and death camp experiences when details of the physical and psychiatric examination reports from reparations applications became public.

PSYCHOANALYTIC INVESTIGATIONS

The classically Freudian theoretical orientation, maintained by many psychoanalysts, seemed insufficient to conceptualize and explain the bewildering array of symptoms presented by the survivors. Freud defined as traumatic any experience breaking through a person's "stimulus barrier."[31] He stressed that the term "traumatic" refers to a temporary condition: Having suffered trauma for a brief period, one returns to a relatively unthreatened state.[32] This definition, based on acute, singular events, could not apply to the months, and even years, of daily degradation and an almost certain death. The Holocaust brought forth a new reality, totally at variance with the social and moral framework formerly taken for granted.

Classical psychoanalytic theory provided three models for the understanding of psychopathology: trauma, which emphasized the undermining of psychic functioning by external forces; developmental arrest, manifesting itself in fixations at certain stages of psychic development, or in the stunted development of certain coping functions (ego); and intrapsychic conflict, an inability to resolve internal (usually unconscious) conflicts. While these three processes operate in isolation, at times they can combine and interweave, allowing trauma to influence both developmental arrest and intrapsychic conflict.

Psychiatrists who disagreed with Freud cited the traumatic neuroses, first observed in World War I, as proof that danger to self-preservation (in contrast to psychosexual conflicts) can be a cause of neurosis. Refuting this criticism, Freud stated, "It would seem highly improbable that a neurosis would come into being because of objective presence of danger, without any participation of the deeper levels of the mental apparatus."[33] Since then, traumatic conditions have been defined as "any conditions which seem definitely unfavorable, noxious, or drastically injurious to the development of the young individual."[34] This definition omits the possibility of trauma having a psychologically deleterious effect on adults. The view that "[e]xternal traumas are turned into internal ones if they touch on, coincide with, or symbolize the fulfillment of either deep-seated anxieties or wish fantasies" is also restricted.[35] These perspectives were difficult to reconcile with the observations of the symptoms of Holocaust survivors.

At the time of the examinations for the reparations program, physicians struggled to determine what constitutes a trauma, particularly in instances of late-appearing sequelae. Comparable psychoanalytic data were lacking (regarding an institutionally sanctioned master plan for the deliberate extinction of a group of people who were regarded as unfit to inhabit the earth with other humans), despite existing historical evidence of tragedies involving attempted genocide. The claim that survivors of other man-made and natural disasters may show symptoms resembling those suffered by Holocaust survivors requires further investigation.[36]

At this time, there is little disagreement that a sudden, acute event can breach the stimulus barrier, overwhelm the psychic apparatus, and render the victim helpless for a time. To understand the varying impact of the traumatic event on different individuals, the meaning of the stimulus and the relationship of the traumatic event to the phases of individual development must be considered on a case-by-case basis. A little boy at the height of his Oedipal phase, for example, may be more vulnerable to a stimulus symbolizing castration, or a younger child to prolonged parental absence (temporary physical separation or death). Responsible investigators also agree that powerful pathogenic effects can be detected as later sequelae in symptomatic survivors of massive and cumulative assault, even without evidence of pronounced pathological predisposition prior to persecution. Cumulative trauma can be extreme trauma resulting in permanent psychological changes.[37]

Clinical illustrations demonstrate that persistent and intense trauma can damage optimal adaptive function and that such effects on parents may affect members of the second generation in survivor families.[38] A young man told his therapist that during his childhood, when he misbehaved, his mother placed his head in the kitchen oven, warning him that this was what Nazis did to Jews in concentration and death camps during the Holocaust. Another patient reported that his mother frequently reminisced about her Auschwitz experiences, describing them as if they had been merry adventures, akin to romping in the fields at a summer vacation resort with girlfriends from her home town. Even though survivors' fantasies of halcyon rescue and reunion with friends and relatives are considered adaptive attempts to sustain themselves during life *in extremis*, treating such fantasies as reasonable, accurate memories (related by a mother to her young son) may indicate possible disturbance in the parent and may also impede the development of reality testing in a growing child.

The passage of West German indemnification laws, having provided an impetus for investigating survivors' emotional problems and for reexamining trauma theories, gradually produced reports in psychiatric journals, beginning in the early and middle 1960s, concerning some survivors' psychological problems, including the late effects of persecution. Data were collected largely from surveys, personal interviews, and from the psychotherapeutic treatment of survivor parents.[39]

When, in 1967, the International Psychoanalytic Association Congress in Copenhagen brought Holocaust survivors' problems to international attention, the general tone of the discussion suggested that the traditional psychoanalytic understanding of the effects of trauma lacked certain important elements necessary to understand and treat survivors suffering significant psychological impairment.[40] Symposium participants stressed that permanent injury to the ego—expressed, for instance, in alteration of personal identity or psychosis-like clinical manifestations—and various other major sequelae seemed to substantiate the view that the pretraumatic personality might play only a minor role in the symptoms of a survivor.[41] In any case, if other channels were blocked, the survivor often directed aggression toward off-spring, thus perpetuating the original traumatic impact of the Holocaust.[42] Because of the extreme circumstances in concentration camps—where only survival behavior had meaning and where the difference between life and death was arbitrary and unpredictable—memories often usurped fantasies in the survivors' mental life. Therefore, some symposium participants thought that attempting to reactivate fantasy life might be therapeutic. However, the main work to be done in the treatment of survivors was to help them to mourn.[43]

SURVIVOR SYNDROME

The identification of a group of symptoms as "survivor syndrome" was one landmark in the psychoanalytic study of Holocaust victims.[44] This is not to suggest that the appearance of this syndrome is universal among Holocaust survivors or its symptoms unique or exclusive to them. The manifestations of the survivor syndrome are multiple, varied, and often recognizable by a conglomerate of palpable psychopathological consequences. Observation and study of nearly 1,000 Holocaust victims indicated consistently recurring manifestations: anxiety, chronic depressive states, tendencies for isolation and withdrawal, psychosomatic complaints, and in some extreme cases, an appearance that suggested a similarity to the *muselman* ("living corpse") stage of concentration camp prisoners, whose apathy and hopelessness suggested imminent death. The most prominent complaint cited was anxiety, associated with fears of renewed persecution. The frequently silent and huddled figures who applied for reparations had numerous gastrointestinal and musculo-skeletal complaints. The depressive equivalents encountered by examiners appeared as feelings of fatigue, a sense of heaviness, and emptiness. Disorders of sleep were common and included fear of falling asleep as well as early morning awakening. A number of applicants showed a striking inability to verbalize the traumatic events they had suffered, especially under the circumstances of having to report to an examiner who might be viewed suspiciously as a representative of authority. This compounded the examiner's difficulty in assessing the survivor who presented the often puzzling selective silences.

A haunting aspect of the depression seen in survivor families was an inability to mourn appropriately for relatives killed during the Holocaust. The lack of opportunity for this dubious luxury was a tragic deprivation resulting in later problems. Survivor parents often superimposed their memories of children killed in the Holocaust on children born after the liberation. Survivor parents were passionately protective of their children and responded to the children's mild illnesses more intensely than would an average family or even one where a child had died as a result of illness or accident.

Nevertheless, in recovery, many survivors have shown an unusual degree of psychic strength and resilience, and have adapted to their renewed lives with great vitality. Many have achieved remarkable success and, due to their commitment to continuity and life-affirming attitudes, have inspired their children to be dedicated to a life of responsibility and service.

ROLE OF PRE-HOLOCAUST PATHOLOGY

Clinical data shows that massive, severe, and cumulative trauma may be the most significant determinant in the appearance of late symptoms in survivors, despite an absence of pre-Holocaust predisposition. While the following vignettes of three adolescents captured by the Nazis and taken to a concentration camp bear a certain resemblance to each other, the influence of their pretraumatic personalities on adult psychological symptoms differs significantly.[45]

Susan was a fifty-year-old woman who sought treatment for relief of almost constant feelings of guilt and anxiety. She was a frequent visitor to hospital emergency rooms because of gastrointestinal and cardiovascular complaints. Despite her physicians' advice to stop, she smoked two packs of cigarettes a day. She was married to an American-born man who was bitter and truculent. He attributed his disappointment in life to having to earn his salary at what he regarded as demeaning work, which deprived him of the time and energy to devote to his artistic and creative talents. The couple, living in considerable marital discord, had two grown children. Their elder child, a daughter, was successful in her profession, but was probably bulimic and apparently had severe difficulties in her relationships with men. The patient's younger son indicated some ability to forge a successful career.

The patient, born in a western European capital, is the younger daughter of an affluent Jewish family. At age ten, her entire family, including an older brother, was captured and sent to a concentration camp, where they spent the next four years. All survived except her father, who contracted dysentery and died in the patient's arms a few weeks before American forces liberated the camp. Though the patient rarely spoke to others about her experiences, she did so readily in treatment, describing the horrors of the camp in some detail. There she had almost lost the wish to live another day and felt sustained by the thought that if life became utterly unbearable, the reasonable certainty of imminent death would bring ultimate relief.

Throughout imprisonment, the patient's father was a sustaining force. He was unfailingly involved with his family and retained his optimistic temperament, predicting Allied victories and an end to the persecution. With great sadness she recalled his last days, when he was exhausted with dysentery and pneumonia. She was aware that she had not been able to mourn him adequately. Following her liberation, she returned to her native city with her brother and mother, who remarried soon thereafter. The patient resented her stepfather. After a few years, he died and the family immigrated to the United States. At first cautious in treatment, she later showed increased trust, but continued to employ a somewhat flip and cynical manner, obviously designed to ward off strong affects. She was constantly preoccupied with feelings of guilt and with worries about her children, mother, husband, and dog. She derived her major gratification from work, which she performed with skill and responsibility. In treatment, she frequently made her own interpretations because accepting something from her therapist would place her in his debt. In a similar vein, she consistently paid her bill at the end of each month before receiving a written statement. She also kept meticulous track of the passage of time and halted sessions herself because she could not easily tolerate being dismissed and would much rather control her leaving.

As far as could be determined, the patient's early development never indicated any clear potential for the sustained and chronic disabilities that appeared in her adult life. In many ways, her guilt, self-deprecation, tendency for somatization, reclusiveness, and leanings toward xenophobic attitudes conform to the complex of symptoms often seen as late sequelae in Holocaust survivors. The absence of any convincing history of significant psychopathology before her incarceration suggests that the major contribution to her symptoms derived from her experiences and those of her family during the Holocaust. The age of the patient during her concentration-camp experiences may have rendered her particularly vulnerable, as is often seen in many who were adolescents at the time of their victimization. Furthermore, her extremely close relationship to her dead father and her difficulties in the completion of mourning may well have contributed to an identification with the only member of her family who did not survive and facilitated a self-designation as the obligatory victim in the surviving family.

Occasionally, therapists encounter patients whose pathology may seem to be accounted for by both internal and external circumstances present before the events of the Holocaust, and therefore not inspire a compelling need for further examination of possible trauma-related pathology. This second vignette of a patient, who sought treatment for an unusual perversion, is a case in point.[46] He would seek out a barber who would have the appearance of a stereotypical Nazi and ask to be shaved. Appearing not to be satisfied, he would request repeated and closer shaving, all the while masturbating under the sheet draping his body. Noting the increasing impatience of the barber, the patient would reach a climax and ejaculate as closely as he might coincide with the barber's mounting exasperation.

During his youth, the patient had attended a Polish military school. As the only Jewish student, he was subjected to brutal "hazing" by fellow students, abetted by teachers. As a result, he developed sadistic retaliatory fantasies. World War II began when the patient was in his late teens. His mother and grandmother were killed by the Nazis, and he was separated from his father. Speaking Polish fluently, he was able to "pass" until he was trapped in the Warsaw ghetto, where he became a heroic figure in the uprising against the Nazis. He recalled this period as the only time in his life when he was free of anxiety. The analyst saw the perversion as a situation in which the patient was able to enact a double role as that of a victim and also a master. He considered all the necessary conditions for an explanation of the patient's psychopathology to have antedated the events of the Holocaust. Furthermore, the Warsaw ghetto rebellion allowed the patient to express the retaliatory fantasies he developed during his school days, without any obvious sense of guilt. Therefore, he remained symptom-free at that time, only to develop perverse symptoms after surviving the Holocaust.

A possible alternative view is that the barber, who played such an important role in the perversion, represented more than the antisemitic Polish officers at the military school. He could have represented a displacement from the patient's father of an early childhood period and the Nazis of a later time. The horrors of the Warsaw ghetto, where so many Jews died, might well have been the organizing factor, fixating the perversion. Therefore, the symptom might not have appeared in adult life under ordinary circumstances. The perversion also could be seen as part of a survivor syndrome, representing a reenactment of an exposure to victimization ultimately resulting in a (fantasied) triumph over the Nazis.[47] It was not possible to determine the reason for the choice of this particular symptom, rather than another, but the importance of this clinical vignette is that it illustrates how Holocaust events can become the crucial organizing factors, producing symptoms with an *anlage* in much earlier experiences.

The interwoven strands of unmistakably preexisting pathology and the influence of the Holocaust in determining the final outcome during a survivor's adult life are illustrated by the following situation.[48] A trim and energetic man in his forties was referred by a colleague who had seen the patient and his family for clarification of marital and family problems. The patient indicated a wish to be referred for individual treatment, preferably psychoanalysis. In individual treatment, he described an increasingly consuming jealousy, which focused on a relationship his wife had had years before their marriage. The patient's jealousy was triggered when he came across a book in their home library that was given to his wife years previously and inscribed to her with an affectionate note on the fly leaf. From the moment of seeing the book, the patient was overcome by almost constant thoughts about his wife's previous relationship, embellished with florid fantasies of sexual activities she might have had with her former friend.

The patient described his background in a well-organized way. He was born in an Eastern European *shtetl*, where most of the inhabitants belonged to an ultra-Orthodox Hasidic sect, led by a rigid and authoritarian rabbi. The patient's father, ill for years with a pulmonary disease, had limited capacity to work. When the patient was twelve years old, his father died, leaving the family impoverished and destitute. As was customary, the patient was sent to neighboring families for meals. He was fed dregs and felt like a degraded beggar. Shortly after the father's death, the patient's younger sister took ill and died of a poorly defined infectious disease.

For months after the father's funeral, the grieving boy was troubled by dreams peopled by demonic figures. The patient appeared to have some difficulty in finding the appropriate English expression to identify these figures. The therapist, attempting a clarification, used the Hebrew phrase for "Angel of Death," whereupon the patient smiled in recognition and commented with some surprise that the analyst knew the Hebrew term.

By the time the patient was thirteen, the Nazis had overrun the area where the patient lived, his mother and he were captured, herded into a boxcar, and sent to Auschwitz. Having been separated from his mother by the infamous selection process, never to see her again, he cried incessantly for a number of days, until he attained some degree of composure.

In describing life in the concentration camp, the patient tended to gloss over the brutalization and dehumanization to which he was exposed. Instead, he focused his antagonism and mistrust on many of his fellow prisoners. He admired those with leftist affiliations because they had a strong sense of group morale and *esprit de corps*. Months later, the patient was transferred to a labor camp where he felt the commandant was singularly lenient. The discrepancy between his hostility toward his fellow prisoners (which resembled those directed toward neighbors in his native town) was puzzling in that it contrasted so obviously with his relatively benign attitude toward his Nazi persecutors. After his liberation he joined a Zionist group, made his way to Israel, and worked on a kibbutz for several years before immigrating to the United States. His Zionist sympathies certainly seem to suggest that his contemptuous attitude toward his fellow Jewish concentration-camp inmates was not necessarily based on a generalized Jewish self-hatred, but on other factors—perhaps the frequently occurring identification with the aggressor as a mechanism for coping in the concentration camp. In the United States he studied, entered a business, married, and appeared to embark on his renewed life with energy and enthusiasm. Some lingering bitterness remained about his past, directed mainly against his former life in the *shtetl*. His ever-present wariness and suspicion erupted acutely when he discovered the book his wife's former friend had given her.

His mistrust soon crystallized into a formidable resistance against treatment. He was acquainted with the psychoanalytic procedure, but expressed reluctance about using the couch and insisted on prolonging face-to-face contact. He expressed reservations about each of the several therapists he had previously consulted and was convinced that one female analyst sat in her chair in a most seductive manner. He also expressed sharply polarized attitudes about me, commending me for being reasonably intelligent and humane, but doubtful whether my intellect and skill were sufficient to help him cope with his problems. Besides, he found it distasteful that I seemed "too Jewish" and thought there were too many books and pictures in my office that dealt with Jewish themes. He acknowledged, however, that the items he saw might have reminded him of his childhood community where he felt treated with such contempt. He also wondered whether psychological treatment was what he required, and he wanted more time to think before he committed himself to being analyzed.

Soon after, the patient developed severe tearing of his eyes and coryzal symptoms (nasal mucus), which he attributed to allergies. He said it was not possible to use the couch under such uncomfortable circumstances. Because he had just told me of the separation from his mother at the gates of Auschwitz and the subsequent disconsolate crying, I asked if it were possible that his symptoms might be connected to feelings about the memories he had just described. Although he had previously complained that I listened too much and spoke too little, he now rebuked me for jumping to premature conclusions. On the following day, he arrived for his appointment with dry mucous membranes. He smiled and said sarcastically that the pollen count must have dropped precipitously.

A short time later, the patient told of a recent dream in which he was standing on a rock in a barren place. The surrounding landscape was bleak and forbidding. Off to one side, he noticed buildings that looked like those of a concentration camp. The patient was convinced there were Nazi patrols nearby, in the process of rounding up Jews, and if he did not leave, he would be captured. But he hesitated because the surrounding area was so threatening that he felt it was preferable to allow himself to be taken prisoner. He said he was perplexed by the dream and unable to associate to it. I suggested that committing himself to be captured might also be related to a wish to be reunited with his mother. He promised to consider the analyst's comments and returned the next day to tell me that the dream he had reported was not a recent one. It dated to the time he and his family were seeing the referring psychiatrist, who had given him a more sensible interpretation, but one he could not recall. When the patient was then asked what came to his mind about his apparent need to plan and then execute a test of his current analyst, he angrily reproached me for calling him a liar and told me he would terminate his treatment.

The foundering of the treatment process was attributable to the patient's sensitivity to humiliation and to his fears of intrusion and penetration, as well as to the therapist's possibly premature interpretations. This case confronts us with the challenge of assessing the patient's personal and familial pathology and comparing its influence with that induced, accentuated, or organized by Holocaust experiences.[49] As was previously indicated, a mass of clinical evidence suggested that victims persecuted during their earlier years may be more vulnerable to suffering from later sequelae than those exposed to traumatic events as adults.[50]

CONCLUSION

Although antisemitism and xenophobia have manifested themselves in various forms during the course of Western history, mass murder on the order of the Holocaust is unprecedented. The trauma inflicted upon the Jews of Europe during the Nazi regime was so severe that it left its mark even on persons who had been free of physical and psychological pathologies prior to their victimizations. In one case presented here, pretraumatic morbid tendencies merged with the symptoms of the trauma sustained subsequently.

Silence was a postwar phenomenon observed in many survivors who wished to forget and in those who became aware that their listeners did not wish to know about the horrors. Survivors often neglected their psychic disturbances, their memories, and their mourning as they assiduously attended to their physical needs and the rebuilding of their lives. After a period of latency, defenses gave way and some working-through of the psychological sequelae of the Holocaust trauma became possible. For the most part, these traumatized people displayed an astonishing, hope-inspiring resilience.

NOTES

1. Elie Wiesel, "The Holocaust: Three Views," *ADL Bulletin* (November 1977): 6.

2. Lucy S. Dawidowicz, *The War Against the Jews, 1933–1945* (New York: Holt, Rinehart & Winston, 1976).

3. The use of the term "Holocaust" suggests to some people that the Jewish people have a need to collaborate in their own victimization. Those who are offended by the term remind us that the chronicles and liturgical poetry of the period of the First Crusade (1095–1099) evoke the image of the *Akedah*, the binding for the sacrifice of Isaac, as the antecedent of later Jewish ordeals and hence as a rationalization for them. One important difference must be underscored: Whichever way the story is interpreted, the life of Isaac was spared and human sacrifice was abjured and replaced by animal sacrifice.

4. Y. H. Yerushalmi, personal communication, 1990.

5. Sigmund Freud, "Why War?" (1932), in *The Standard Edition of the Complete Psychological Works of Sigmund Freud* (London: The Hogarth Press, 1964), 22:214–15, was his answer to a question brought up by Einstein in a letter to Freud of July 30, 1932 (22:201).

6. The segment of the Jewish community committed to a monotheistic worship was unrelenting in displaying hostility and antagonism toward worshipers of pagan

deities. There is ample evidence that the Hebrew tribes did not accept monotheism overnight in their adoption of so-called Mosaic law, but worshiped their pagan deities side by side with their newly found monotheism. The monotheistic position finally prevailed after the return from the Babylonian exile and the Persian and Macedonian conquests.

7. St. John Chrysostom, St. Augustine, and St. Ambrose

8. Despite the Christian view that the crucifixion and sacrifice of Jesus was considered necessary for the salvation of the world, it was also employed as a projection onto Judas and the Jews in general. The projective aspect is evident in the gospels. For example, the Eucharist renewed in a symbolic form the sacrifice of children, which had been abjured in Judaism and made necessary the myth that Jews use the blood of Christian children to prepare matzoh for Passover. The Gospels of Mark and John state quite clearly: "His blood be on us and on our children." This statement establishes the theme of "blood libel," which later became a central, dark, and ominous core of anti-Jewish feelings.

9. Although the true murderer of a Christian boy was known to the police, a Jew, Mendel Beilis, of Kiev, was accused by the Union of the Russian People in 1911 of having killed him for ritual purposes. For two years the police cooperated with the Minister of Justice to assemble false testimonies. With the help of excellent lawyers and the revolutionary press, the Minister of Justice was exposed as having staged the trial. Beilis was acquitted, but the blood libel itself was not officially rescinded. The Beilis trial represented the Russian struggle over the "Jewish question," as well as the conflict between the regime and the "radical public opinion." H. H. Ben-Sasson, *A History of the Jewish People* (Cambridge, Mass.: Harvard University Press, 1976), 888.

10. Jacob Arlow, personal communication, 1989, maintains that clinical observations alone may lead to certain conclusions about individual psychopathology related to antisemitism, yet leave in question the meanings and causes of the pervasive societal manifestations leading to the Holocaust.

11. Joseph Cultreara, personal communication, 1990.

12. John H. Hanson, "Nazi Culture: The Social Uses of Fantasy as Repression," in *Psychoanalytic Reflections on the Holocaust: Selected Essays*, ed. S. A. Luel and Paul Marcus (New York: Ktav, 1984).

13. Robert J. Lifton, "Medicalized Killing in Auschwitz," in *Psychoanalytic Reflections on the Holocaust: Selected Essays*, ed. S. A. Luel and Paul Marcus (New York: Ktav, 1984).

14. Mortimer Ostow, "The Psychodynamics of Apocalyptic: Discussions of Papers on Identification with the Nazi Phenomenon," *International Journal of Psychoanalysis* 67 (1986): 277–85.

15. Ibid.

16. During the two centuries before and after the beginning of the Common Era, many apocalypses appeared in the Middle East, perhaps in response to Greek and Roman conquests. The ones begun by Jews were probably adopted by the Christian community. Official religious communities tended to frown upon them; the Jewish canon accepted no apocalypses, and only the Revelation of John was accepted into the Christian canon. Features of various apocalypses differed, each designed to respond to local conditions. They represent in general a dualistic quality where two forces are in a cosmic struggle with each other. The forces of evil are led by a demon

and at first prevail; ultimately they are crushed by the forces of good, led by a messianic figure. The evil in the world then is replaced by a messianic era, 1,000 years of prosperity in the Christian tradition.

17. It must be emphasized that the official church tended to discourage apocalyptic thinking, but it nevertheless continued to engage interest. Fantasy gave way to activism during the fifth century of the Common Era and foreshadowed the adventurism of the Crusades, which enveloped Europe during the Middle Ages.

18. This formulation is suggested in a hypothetical and speculative sense and only as one possible factor that must be studied further in relation to historical data to establish any degree of validation.

19. Ostow, "Psychodynamics of Apocalyptic."

20. Jews are enjoined to remember the Exodus after their enslavement in Egypt at every Passover, and the destruction of the Temple in Jerusalem followed by their scattering to the Diaspora, as well as other events of persecution and suffering.

21. Aharon Appelfeld, "One Guiding and Abiding Feeling," *Hadoar*, September 1978.

22. Ernst Kris, "The Recovery of Childhood Memories in Psychoanalysis," in *The Psychoanalytic Study of the Child*, 53 vols. (New York: International Universities Press, 1956), 11:54–88.

23. E. Rappaport, "Beyond Traumatic Neurosis," *International Journal of Psychoanalysis* 49 (1968): 720.

24. Wiesel, "The Holocaust," 5.

25. Paul Friedman, "The Road Back for the D.P.'s," *Commentary* 6 (1948): 502–10; idem, "Some Aspects of Concentration Camp Psychology," *American Journal of Psychiatry* 105 (1949): 601–5.

26. Miriam Williams and Judith S. Kestenberg, "Introduction and Discussion in Workshop on Children of Survivors," summarized in *Journal of the American Psychoanalytic Association* 22 (1974): 91–100.

27. Milton Kestenberg, "Discriminatory Aspects of the German Indemnification Policy: A Continuation of Persecution," in *Generations of the Holocaust*, ed. Martin S. Bergmann and Milton E. Jucovy (New York: Basic Books, 1982), 67–79. He wrote about K. Kisker, a distinguished German psychiatrist, whose influence prompted the German courts to revise their usual view and rule in favor of restitution for psychiatric reasons.

28. Kestenberg, "Discriminatory Aspects," has written eloquently on some of the problems that attended the application of the reparations law passed by the Federal German Republic. Almost immediately questions arose centering on the complicated procedures involved in making a claim and in the process of filing the application. Under paragraph seven of the law, compensation can be refused for inaccurate statements, even when made only for simplification in the presentation of evidence.

29. Ibid.

30. Cited by M. Kestenberg concerning his client.

31. Freud, "Beyond the Pleasure Principle" (1920), *Standard Edition*, 18:3–64, spoke of an excitation from outside that is powerful enough to break through the protective shield. This is actually a metapsychological assumption and not, strictly speaking, a clinical observation that rests on a series of assumptions that, in turn, are also based on abstract and unverifiable laws. One such law, for example, would be that the human organism is equipped with an apparatus to protect the individual

from overstimulation. Another such law would hold that this hypothetical apparatus can function only within a certain range of stimuli; if it is subjected to a massive dose of stimuli, the barrier will break down and a state of shock and disorganization will ensue.

32. Freud, "Introductory Lectures" (1916), *Standard Edition*, 15–16: 15–463.

33. Freud, "Inhibitions, Symptoms and Anxiety" (1926), *Standard Edition*, 20: 77–175 quote cited on 129. Theorizing that there is nothing in the "unconscious" that corresponds to the annihilation of life, Freud continued, "I am therefore, inclined to adhere to the view that the fear of death should be regarded as analogous to the fear of castration." More important was Freud's recognition of a certain sense of abandonment "by the superego powers of destiny, so that there are no longer any safeguards against danger." Ibid., 20: 130.

34. Phyllis Greenacre, "The Influence of Infantile Trauma on Genetic Patterns," in *Emotional Growth: Psychoanalytic Studies of the Gifted and a Great Variety of Other Individuals*, 2 vols. (New York: International Universities Press, 1971), 1:277.

35. Anna Freud, "Comments on Trauma," in *Psychic Trauma*, ed. S. Furst (New York: Basic Books, 1967), 241.

36. This claim has frequently been regarded as a trivialization of the Holocaust. Argument about such a question misses the point. All human suffering is deplorable and should not be subjected to rivalry. Each tragedy has its special qualities, and objective scientific investigation is best utilized in the service of gaining increased knowledge about their particular characteristics and aftereffects.

37. Ilse Grubrich-Simitis, "Extreme Traumatization as Cumulative Trauma," *Psychoanalytic Study of the Child*, 53 vols. (New Haven, Conn.: Yale University Press, 1981), 36:415–50, has summed up this point of view in discussing extreme trauma, which can become cumulative trauma and thus cause permanent, rather than only temporary, changes in the psychic apparatus, even in the apparent absence of any predisposition. She pointed out that the threat of narcissistic depletion in these instances was due not only to extended periods of deprivation of external supplies, but also to superego changes derived from massive assaults on the victim's psyche. These changes consist of regression to archaic forms of superego functioning and sometimes led to severe changes in the ego ideal. The devalued image, promoted by the persecutors and felt excruciatingly by the victim, became insidiously established in the ideal self of the victim. It is paradoxical and tragic that this process occurred by way of the very mechanism, identification with the aggressor, that had been utilized originally by victims to stem the tide of hopelessness and to check the process of narcissistic depletion. Aside from the effects of superego functioning and the changes in the ego ideal that have been noted, there were also effects on ego functioning in those persecuted and traumatized. In many instances, the effects were lasting and not always subtle.

38. Milton E. Jucovy, "Telling the Holocaust Story: A Link Between the Generations," *Psychoanalytic Inquiry* 5 (1985): 31–49.

39. Several of these pioneer efforts should be mentioned, but they cannot all be noted in this introduction. William G. Niederland, "The Problem of the Survivor," *Journal of the Hillside Hospital* 10 (1961): 233–47; idem, "Clinical Observations on the 'Survivor Syndrome': Symposium in Psychic Traumatization Through Social Catastrophe," *International Journal of Psychoanalysis* 49 (1968): 313–15, was one of the earliest to study defenses employed against the stresses of life in concentration

camps and to describe the psychiatric disorders that appeared both early and late. Paul Chodoff, "Late Effects of the Concentration Camp Syndrome," *Archives of General Psychiatry* (1963): 22–23, described some of the late effects of the concentration-camp syndrome, as did Leo Eitinger, "Pathology of the Concentration Camp Syndrome," *Archives of General Psychiatry* (1961): 371–79, in Norway. He drew a harrowing picture of the prisoners' terror and helplessness and the physical cruelty to which they were subjected. Henry Krystal, ed., *Massive Psychic Trauma* (New York: International Universities Press, 1968), edited a volume on massive psychic trauma, which drew together many of the observations of the early pioneers who became involved in the study of survivors. H. Zvi Winnik, "Psychiatric Disturbances of Holocaust Survivors: Symposium of the Israel Psychoanalytic Society," *Israel Annals of Psychiatry and Related Disciplines* 5 (1967): 91–100, who had chaired a symposium sponsored by the Israel Psychoanalytic Society in 1966, reported on the psychopathology and treatment of victims of Nazi persecution.

40. Proceedings from "Psychic Traumatization through Social Catastrophe," International Psychoanalytic Association Congress, Copenhagen, 1967. Participants from several countries attended this symposium, including Erich Simenauer, H. Zvi Winnik, William Niederland, Emmanuel de Wind, Martin Wangh, and Klaus D. Hoppe.

41. When problems of technique were discussed at the symposium, analysts differed about the relative significance they would assign to the roles of abreaction, insight, efforts at reconstruction, the recovery of childhood memories, and the analysis of the transference. The discussion developed no general consensus about which category or modality of technique might prove most helpful. De Wind stressed assisting the survivor in dealing with aggression, on the basis of his belief that warded-off aggression was behind both the prevalence of chronic depression as well as the frequency of somatic illness among survivors.

42. E. de Wind, "The Confrontation with Death," *International Journal of Psychoanalysis* 49 (1968): 302–5.

43. Martin Wangh, "A Psychogenetic Factor in the Recurrence of War: Symposium on Psychic Traumatization through Social Catastrophe," *International Journal of Psychoanalysis* 49 (1968): 319–23.

44. Niederland, "Clinical Observations on the 'Survivor Syndrome.' "

45. Milton E. Jucovy, "Prelude," in *Generations of the Holocaust*, ed. Martin S. Bergmann and Milton E. Jucovy (New York: Basic Books, 1982), 3–29.

46. Abraham Freedman, "Psychoanalytic Study of an Unusual Perversion," *Journal of the American Psychoanalytic Association* 26 (1978): 749–78, and Harold P. Blum, "Discussion of 'Psychoanalytic Study of an Unusual Perversion,' " *Journal of the American Psychoanalytic Association* 26 (1978): 785–92.

47. Blum, "Discussion."

48. Jucovy, "Prelude."

49. The patient's symptoms and behavior patterns suggested a glaring propensity for projection, verging on a paranoid state. This patient could have been exposed to homosexual seduction during his imprisonment. The gratuitous reference to the kindness of the commandant of the labor camp provokes some curiosity about this possibility, but there was no opportunity to explore it further. If such exposures did indeed occur to a sensitive adolescent, they might have rekindled earlier feelings of humiliation and exploitation beyond the usual suffering endured during later perse-

cution. It did seem quite clear that this man had a need not to be understood too easily or quickly, perhaps based on fears of intrusion and penetration. Premature attempts to foster a therapeutic alliance by making clarifying remarks, such as the one about the Angel of Death and later attempts to explore his coryzal symptoms may have been counterproductive.

50. Editor's note [CK]: Dr. Jucovy's second patient who acted out his pains and conflicts in a structured symptom, akin to a perversion, was vulnerable to developing psychic problems as a result of pre-Holocaust experiences. In contrast, the first patient, who seemed to be relatively free of pretraumatic vulnerabilities, presented characterological problems instead of symptoms. The third patient's jealousy and sensitivity to "intrusion" can be seen as a combination of specific symptoms and a more generalized personality characteristic. Similarly, many of the diagnostic criteria for posttraumatic stress disorder are clearly pervasive, characterological markers of ego impairment, such as detachment, estrangement, restricted range of affect, hypervigilance, and "distress or impairment in social, occupational, or other important areas of functioning," such as cognition or reality testing, for example (as noted in American Psychiatric Association, *Diagnostic and Statistical Manual of Mental Disorders*, 4th. [Washington, D.C.: The American Psychiatric Association, 1994], 428–29). These reactions are quite different from such symptoms as agoraphobia (associated with panic disorder), exhibitionism, pathological gambling, or pyromania. The differences in the symptoms can be understood as a reflection of the severity of the trauma and its impact on ego functioning. Therefore, a cluster of distinguishing symptoms indicating an impairment of the body or psychological ego might represent degrees of posttraumatic stress (not a general borderline personality disorder), whereas a specific symptom might be the result of an ego's ability to organize and circumscribe the effects of internal conflict or noxious external influences.

2

Historical Trauma:
Psychohistorical Reflections
on the Holocaust

Robert Prince

A gifted eight year old asked, "Why did the Nazis hate the Jews so much?" After a minute of silent reflection he answered his own question: "Because of their [Jews'] beliefs." Of course, he is completely wrong. Had he asked his question about the Spanish expulsion of Jews in 1492, he might have had a leg to stand on, but for the Nazis, a Jew's beliefs, the contents of a Jew's mind, were totally irrelevant. The Jews of the Grand Inquisitor Torquamada's time in Spain, as terrible as it was, had the opportunity to change the aspect about themselves that was hated, their religion, and could survive and even prosper. Despite brutality, there could be continuity and thus meaning existed. The Jews of Hitler's time were hated for what they *were*, only and entirely for the reason of being racially Jewish—completely, totally, and irrevocably. The Nazis so completely obliterated the humanness of their victims that there was nothing Jews, adults or children, could do to change themselves or to modify that passionate hatred.

This was so incomprehensible to the little boy because it represented a traumatic disruption of his personal world-view. His own experience within his family—that his subjectivity mattered—had produced a framework of personal meanings that was threatened by his confrontation with history.

History can be thought of as a form of memory. In a social parallel to the personal myth—the memory created to support the repression of trauma—the child's question can be understood as a psychohistorical moment: the ontogenesis of a historical myth, namely that hate, Nazi hate, had meaning.[1]

The underlying theme of this chapter is the struggle between meaning and the attempt to destroy it. To develop this theme, I will review the nature of the trauma that is represented by the Holocaust and examine the new dimensions it introduces to humanity's self-image. In that context, I wish to describe and, to the extent possible, understand a set of overt responses to the Holocaust. Second, I will turn attention to survivors and children of survivors, and their illumination of the nature of traumatic effects.

PERSONAL AND HISTORICAL TRAUMA

The term "trauma" is usually reserved for an overwhelming shock or injurious event in an individual's personal development; it may be a single acute stress or a cumulative strain. I have chosen the term "historical trauma" to denote an event of a social nature, occurring in the course of human history, that has an impact both on the development of individual persons and on the further stream of history.

The Holocaust was a historical trauma of great enormity, magnified by the fact that the killers of the Holocaust were not of a barbarous nation, some primitive tribe suddenly empowered. The Holocaust was not like the massacre of thousands of Armenian peasants by Ottoman troops in 1894, nor like the Turkish soldiers who drove men, women, and children into the Iranian desert, killing hundreds of thousands, in 1915. These "horrible butcheries came as a shock to a Europe unused to such violence, and were blamed entirely on the exceptional barbarity of the terrible Turk."[2] The perpetrators were the Germans. Notwithstanding their traditions of music, science, art, and philosophy, which represented western civilization at its height, and which earned them high regard as the most cultivated and disciplined people in Europe, the historical record is absolutely clear: They and their institutions enthusiastically, passionately, embraced Hitler and his aims.[3]

In a speech at Obersalzburg on August 22, 1939, Hitler, more barbarous than a primitive tribal head, proclaimed, "Our strength is in our quickness and brutality. . . . Thus, for the time being I have sent to the east only Death's Head units, with orders to kill without pity or mercy all men, women, and children of Polish race or language."[4] Thus, the Holocaust represents a "historical novum" in that "previous boundaries and assumptions about human nature and the nature of history were destroyed."[5] The Holocaust "has challenged our conventional social, cultural, and psychological criteria of analysis and interpretation primarily because it has revealed new data about human behavior that require new categories of understanding."[6] It represents the actualization of scientific, technological, and organizational progress as horror. The Holocaust necessitates a restructuring of conceptions of reality and ethics.

HISTORY AND PSYCHOLOGY

The application of the historian's expertise to psychology or the psychoanalyst's expertise to history is required to address the issue of social or historical trauma. However, such endeavors have often been received with much ambivalence. Besides Freud's speculative psychohistorical writing about a primal past, and a few other notable exceptions, there is relatively little in the traditional psychoanalytical literature about the effects of history on the development of the psyche. Rather, in keeping with the predominant psychoanalytic concern for internal events, the emphasis has been on the effect of the human psyche on history. Indeed, "reality" poses special problems in psychoanalytic thinking not only because of the general epistemological issues involved, but because in psychoanalysis "reality" often means "psychic reality," which is an intrapersonal experience rather than an external, observable event. Thus the Freudian concept of trauma stresses the inner event of pre-existing unconscious wishes, reverberating to the external stimuli. Establishing what is "formative" about outer, historical events runs contrary to this major thrust.[7]

The world in which psychoanalysis as a discipline unfolded may not have been a stable one, yet certainly a stable world-view prevailed, such that "people of intelligence and good will . . . could take [a certain order] for granted." And an implicit consensus prevailed that the impinging impact of reality "could be subsumed under the apt phrase . . . of the 'average expectable environment.' "[8] In retrospect it is evident that this stability is illusory and may account for the fact that "[a]fter three-fourths of a century, the actual results of psychoanalytic study of history are disappointing."[9]

On the part of historians, there seems to be conflict and wariness about embracing psychology. Jacques Barzun warns against "the attempt to rescue Clio from pitiable maidenhood by artificial insemination."[10] However, William Langer presents a different perspective. He exhorts historians to "be particularly concerned with the problem whether major changes in the psychology of a society or culture can be traced, even in part, to some severe trauma suffered in common—that is, with the question whether whole communities, like individuals, can be profoundly affected by some shattering experience. If it is indeed true that every society or culture had a 'unique psychological fabric,' deriving at least in part from past common experiences and attitudes, it seems reasonable to suppose that any great crisis, such as famine, pestilence, natural disaster, or war, should leave its mark on the group, the intensity and duration of the impact depending, of course, on the nature and magnitude of the crisis" and the diverse reactions of the individual group members. "[T]hese varying responses are apt to be reflected chiefly in the immediate effects of the catastrophe. Over the long term it seems likely that the group would react in a manner most nearly corresponding to the underlying requirements of the majority of its members—in other words, that despite great variations as between individuals there would be a dominant attitudinal pattern."[11]

The nature of the Holocaust trauma precludes any consensus about reality. The importance of the "intensity of stimuli" in the causation of trauma cannot be denied, but the "challenge to the integrity of one's self stems from [the interplay between] the meaning of the event and resulting affective responses."[12] It is well known, for example, that the traumatic effects of personal catastrophe are greater when the source is a human agency as opposed to a disaster in nature. This phenomenon can be understood only on the basis of the implied meanings. Moreover, it is the meaning of trauma that determines the psychological consequence.

Psychoanalysis, defined by its concern with meanings, has struggled in particular with the meaning of trauma. The classical position holds that external, reality events have their traumatic effects precisely because of their resonance with preexisting intrapsychic themes. Resulting symptoms are therefore understood to be products of psychic processes, ultimately symbolizing unconscious contents. However, massive trauma destroys the ability to symbolize and disrupts the personality organization. Consequently, in the case of massive trauma, a traumatic neurosis occurs, "its symptoms, including traumatic dreams," not amenable to interpretation. In other words, traumatic neurosis has no unconscious meaning and the capacity for "metaphorization" has been reduced.[13]

SYMBOLIZATION AND METAPHORIZATION

Concentration camp inmates lived in a world beyond, or even before, metaphor where behavior had no symbolic meaning.[14] The task of seeking "some symbolic realization" may fall on the child of survivors, whose own "symptoms may express metaphorical attempts at such a re-creation and restitution of the parent's symbolic processes."[15] Multiple meanings can be condensed into narrow symptom-channels in the form of some Holocaust-related obsession or symptom. Each traumatic image can have multiple meanings and reverberations in the person's inner world, and each of the particular meanings can remain fluid over time without losing any strength. Because the powerful impact of the Holocaust is interpreted and processed by unique individuals, it fails to have a common significance for either survivors or their children. Meanings may also be altered and developed by events subsequent to the trauma and, therefore, have great bearing on the clinical sequelae.

Within this paradigm, repetition, a phenomenon almost universally associated with the diagnosis of posttraumatic stress disorder (PTSD), can be understood in two ways. First, it can represent an attempt at mastery, an effort to impose order where meaning has broken down. Alternatively, repetitions in the form of traumatic reexperiencing, such as concretization of the trauma via flashbacks, manifest a failure of symbolization and the inability to integrate the trauma into a system of representations. These emotionally intense experiences are thus closely related to their phenomenological opposite, the state of affect depletion characterized as "psychic numbing."[16] The condition of psychic numbing is among the most important consequences of traumata of the magnitude of the Holocaust. Psychic numbing is described as a posttraumatic effect characterized by detached feelings, estrangement from others, and the loss or decrease in emotional experience.[17] This "psychic closing off" also involves aspects of isolation of affect, denial, and perhaps rationalizations. However, its essence is that it attacks meaning and symbolic functions.[18]

Thus, the effects of trauma can be understood as a function of a system of meanings and as the tension between meaning and its destruction.

MEANINGS, MEMORIES, AND CONTINUITY

The meanings created by the themes introduced into human history by the Holocaust influence many individuals' psychic structure and shape the content of their character. Many concentration camp survivors (and populations in Asia, the Middle East, and the Balkans, who more recently lived through historical trauma) are engaged in the struggle between finding meaning and experiencing numbing. In many cases, their trauma has been transmitted across generational lines to their children.

In post-Holocaust history, survivorhood of the Holocaust is a universal condition of all people. The post-Holocaust population has to suffer the traumatic effects of its new historical themes and the widespread instinctual overload arising from twentieth-century images of annihilation. Phenomena as disparate as the incidence of serial murder and the graphic displays of gore and violence in movies may well be a Holocaust-induced expression of a change in the intensity human beings now require to cross their sensory threshold. One murder and a little blood just doesn't do it anymore. While the defensive regression into a culture of narcissism may be one response to these prevailing conditions, paradoxically, this also seems to be an era of the "victim."[19]

Moreover, indications of global disillusionment and cynicism about ideals, belief systems, and leaders, paralleled by an increasing popularity of fundamentalist religious movements, suggest that post-Holocaust humanity expresses alternately a new nihilism and a fear of a violent, intolerant deity—finding apocalypse in both. Altogether, these phenomena point to the recursive effects of existing historical contexts on future social-historical events, which, in turn, create a new context for still later events. In this sense, the aftermath of World War I was the context spawning Nazism and the Holocaust; the violence and terror of those events then affected history, such that today a defended and jaded population seeks greater intensity of stimulation while simultaneously embracing and rejecting established belief systems.

The task of identifying the effects of Holocaust meanings is an enormously complex one. Above all, the Holocaust was an event of awesome magnitude, one in which the very best of human behavior—endurance, heroism, and sacrifice—was displayed along with the very worst. Understanding the effects of the Holocaust on present social currents is complicated in that perpetrators of the violence and murder, bystanders who allowed it to take place, and victims have much in common.[20] Furthermore, as is true for traumatized individuals, group and national memories, too, are subject to repression and distortion. The recent historical revisionism is an example. The grosser claims—that the Holocaust is a historical fabrication, the gas chambers Jewish propaganda, and that the Allies treated German prisoners of war just as badly as Germans treated the Jews—are readily discounted. Nevertheless, these assertions do facilitate more subtle distortions—for example, the denial of the centrality of antisemitism in the Jewish experience—and result in renewed manifestations of antisemitism in Europe, in certain sectors in the United States, and probably in other countries as well. The social phenomenon of revisionism has a direct parallel in individual repression of traumatic memories, resulting in symptom formation and in distortions of the ability to perceive and test reality.

Ironically, many of the groups that had key roles in the perpetration of Holocaust crimes have come forward to claim a place in the victim ranks. Thus, Austria elected Kurt Waldheim as its leader and presented itself to the world as Hitler's "first victim." Chancellor Kohl of the Federal Republic of Germany invited President Reagan to heal the wounds by laying a wreath at Bitburg—not at Dachau. More recently, the government of Lithuania has issued certificates of exoneration to war criminals, recasting them as nationalist heroes who defended their homeland against Russian aggression.

Truth, Winston Churchill said, is a fragile thing. It requires a bodyguard of lies. In individual psychoanalytic work, the way into complexity is sometimes by way of uncovering distortions. The same method can be applied to the problem of the Holocaust by examining a number of myths that have wide currency.

MYTHS

In the sense that early, incomplete, and sometimes erroneous explanations of Holocaust survivors' psychological dynamics and social behaviors were accepted uncritically, they have become myths. Five such myths will be explored here: passivity, silence, pathology, guilt, and defense.

Passivity

The first of the psychohistorical Holocaust myths evolved as early as 1943 with the uncritical reception of Bettelheim's report of his own incarceration at Dachau in 1938. For many years, a portrait of the passive, regressed behavior of prisoners who identified with the aggressor dominated the conception of the survivor. Subsequent research has supported a rather different picture, namely that survival was facilitated by maintaining the integrity of one's core self, its meanings and relationships. Bettelheim himself obviously endured by applying his intellectual values and adopting a scientific stance that signified a preservation of the core of his "self."[21]

The important matter of maintaining personal meaning and integrity has been approached from several angles. In contrast to the passive strategy described by Bettelheim, survival was enhanced by countering the Nazi attempt to deprive Jews of their dignity, their spirit, and of their pervasive will to live and learn.[22] Similarly, social involvement and an ability, through fantasy, to maintain ties to a past "good object," that is, an important past relationship, helped inmates to endure the concentration camp conditions.[23] There also seems to have been a connection between staying human and staying alive.[24] Those who survived were described as having maintained their dignity and showing a "talent for life." After their liberation, a majority of survivors were able to recover their capacities and function reasonably effectively despite suffering and loss.[25]

Silence

A second Holocaust myth developed about the silence of the survivor. In fact, many—not all—survivors had a tremendous need (and felt a profound obligation to the dead) to speak. They had, however, very ambivalent listeners. Many survivors described both gross refusals to hear, believe, or understand, as well as more covert resistance, subtle interruptions, and deflections of their narrative. That the Holocaust background of hospitalized children of survivors was omitted from otherwise extensive records is evidence of a lack of empathic understanding even on the part of physicians.[26] Under these conditions, the reputed resistance by survivors and their children to psychotherapy might be attributed in part to their doubt that the essential condition for therapy, that is, the "inner readiness" of the therapist to listen, will be fulfilled.[27] This is in concurrence with the general understanding that the reluctance of a patient to speak may be a function of the empathy of the therapist listener.[28]

Pathology

A third myth has to do with the presumptive universality of the "survivor syndrome" and its extension into the second generation. Labeling the "survivor syndrome" a myth is not to deny profound traumatic effects. Indeed to have endured so much and not have been affected would be an indictment of the individual's humanity.[29]

A closer look at the survivor syndrome reveals that the range of symptoms included in the final psychiatric formulation is so broad as to encompass a textbook of human psychopathology. However, I would not object to the word "complex," which can be differentiated from a "syndrome" by its emphasis on shared psychological dynamics rather than manifest, observable outcomes.[30] In contrast to the recognition of a "complex," the insistence on a standardized syndrome subtly undermines the notion of a highly individual posttraumatic adaptation. It also permits the denial of the existence of posttraumatic effects when uniform effects are not found. Finally, it leads to further inaccurate characterizations of survivors. For example, the conscious rejection of the wish to have children and a low birth rate have been attributed to survivors.[31] Contrasting data indicate not only a higher actual birthrate, but the overwhelming importance of generativity to survivor families.[32] Similarly, Milton and Judith S. Kestenberg movingly explore the survivors' response to the Nazi attempt to undermine generativity for all time.[33]

Guilt

"Survivor guilt" is another notion that has a central place in the mythology of survival. The concept emphasizes guilt for the actuality or the presumed widespread fantasy of having survived at the expense of others.[34] By extension, it is also guilt for the actualization of one's own aggression. I have not been impressed by the existence of pervasive survivor guilt, neither during direct interviews with survivors nor in portrayals of survivor parents by their children. One survivor's response to a mental health professional's question about survivor guilt was, "What the hell do I have to be guilty about?"[35] While "survival guilt" undoubtedly does exist as a very complex phenomenon, its actual significance may differ markedly from what has been imputed to it. For example, the guilt may represent an attempt to maintain both personal continuity and ties with lost objects.[36]

Myths as Defense

How can these psychohistorical myths be understood? Above all, they represent an ambivalence about allowing true knowledge of the Holocaust into consciousness. As with personal myths, false memories are created to conceal knowledge that would undermine our sense of reality, self-esteem, and safety. Both personal myths and psychohistorical myths represent compromises. They tend to conceal information, perceptions, and interpretations of the self and the world that would undermine the defensive barriers between the person and the disrupting, traumatizing patterns of meaning embedded in Holocaust images and events.

The Holocaust myths also serve to distance us from identification with the victim. They blunt the trauma of witnessing. By perpetuating the fantasy of the essential otherness of the survivor, we can disavow the possibility of being victimized ourselves and then assert that our own world is safe. There is magical potency in the formula "It can't happen here, not to me and mine, because it belongs to them, there." A special derivative of the flight from identification is the denial of individuality, the negation of personal experience. Often this occurs when the individual meaning is drowned in a collective sea of statistics.

Our internalized values make it almost impossible to accept the blamelessness of the victim of persecution. It is virtually intolerable not to impute at least a slight responsibility to the victim and thereby to remove it from the perpetrator. Thus, we attempt to restore order to the moral universe and to contribute to a delusion of personal control. Further, by blaming the victim, however subtly, we are freed of any moral obligation to make meaningful reparation, and are protected from any guilt incurred by identifying with the aggressor. Myths protect us from what we do not want to know, including just how much blame there is or how far it goes—in our direction!

CHILDREN OF SURVIVORS

In contrast to these psychohistorical myths, which tend to mass characterizations, the data gathered from work with children of survivors demonstrates the profound, diverse effects of the Holocaust trauma. Each of these was colored, albeit in a unique way, by both Holocaust images and family experiences.[37]

In the context of Holocaust imagery mediated by parental experiences, not shared common traits, a complex of developmental themes unfolded, notably issues of trust and mistrust. The trust-mistrust questions are reflected in composite images of the parent in current family reality and of human nature as reflected by human behavior during the Holocaust era. In each case, the rupture of trust in the social order was evoked by historical imagery; yet this rupture reverberated to the patterns of a lasting trust in the family order. The variations on the themes, provided both by history and the family, were vast and were repeated for every major human issue: separation and autonomy, anger and control, shame and grandiosity, anxiety and satisfaction of needs.

That the children of survivors were consciously identified with, or attributed importance to the family Holocaust background, was revealed in their personality styles; preferred modes of interpersonal relationships with parents and others; their Jewish identification; and attitudes, ideas, and beliefs in general, as well as about the Holocaust in particular. This observation is closely related to the process of "transposition," which states that children of survivors live out a deceased family member's life simultaneously with their own. That is, they transpose the past onto the present.[38]

While dramatic contrasts among the children of survivors could be shown on multiple dimensions, two characteristics did seem to prevail almost universally: They have a sense of always having known of their parents' survivorhood, and they want to pass on knowledge of the Holocaust to the next generation. These two common characteristics reflect a struggle for meaning in the face of numbing and an assertion of continuity in the face of the destruction of meaning by the threat of extinction.

Historical Imagery as Organizer of Identity

Historical imagery, mediated by parental experience, can be shown to serve as an unconscious organizer for the identity of children of survivors. For everyone, a sense of reality derives from current surroundings, in part defined by the historical context; the sense of self develops from and is shaped by images absorbed from history as mediated by family and personal experiences. Selectively absorbed historical images can become metaphors for a person's mode of operating in the world and for the core sense of self. When the images are traumatic, the adaptive struggle is between denial and discovery of meanings upon which the self depends for its integrity and vitality.

Such images influence perception in the present, subliminally or directly. For example, a businesswoman was influenced when she rediscovered Holocaust-specific ethical dilemmas in current business decisions. Similarly, a medical student related his emotional experience while preforming a dissection in anatomy class to his understanding of war criminals' habituation to performing acts of horror.

The businesswoman and the medical student were conscious of their fantasies. In every child of a survivor, one can find at least subliminal Holocaust imagery. Detailed inquiry uncovers the invisible threads of history and the disguised fantasies about parents' survival out of which the basic fabric of a person's life is woven. These provide the basic metaphors around which the children of survivors organize their life.

CONCLUSION

In this exposition, person and history, as well as past and present social currents, have shifted between figure and ground. These are mutually influencing forces, not causal, but reciprocal. In circular fashion, the individual is traumatized by events; the traumatized individual affects events. To elucidate this process, the concept of personal myth was applied to the adaptation of individuals, and psychohistorical myth was introduced as an attempted adaptation to traumatic events in historical eras. Similarly, repression and memory in individuals and revisions of the historical record in societies can be compared. Meaning is experienced by individuals, but it inheres in events. In both we find great complexity and thus nonrandom diversity. Both reflect values and goals, moral principles, definitions of boundaries, and a sense of order. And both, of course, can show pathology.

Of utmost importance is the clinical principle, central to psychoanalytic work, that what is not recalled is reenacted.

The child's own answer to his question, "Why did the Nazis hate the Jews so much?" expresses his struggle to adapt to the basic psychological antinomy: love and hate, meaning, and numbing. And this is the struggle of the present historical era.

NOTES

1. Ernst Kris, "The Recovery of Childhood Memories in Psychoanalysis," in *The Psychoanalytic Study of the Child*, 53 vols. (New York: International Universities Press, 1956), 11: 54–88.

2. R. Palmer and Joel Colton, *A History of the Modern World* (New York: Alfred A. Knopf, 1985).

3. Daniel J. Goldhagen, *Hitler's Willing Executioners* (New York: Alfred A. Knopf, 1996).

4. Adolf Hitler, cited by Judith S. Kestenberg and Milton Kestenberg, "The Experience of Survivor Parents," in *Generations of the Holocaust*, ed. Martin S. Bergmann and Milton E. Jucovy (New York: Basic Books, 1982), 54.

5. George Kren, "The Holocaust: Some Unresolved Issues," *Annals of Scholarship* 3 (1984): 39–61.

6. Paul Marcus and Irene Wineman, "Psychoanalysis Encountering the Holocaust," *Psychoanalytic Inquiry* 5 (1985): 85–98.

7. Robert Lifton, "Protean Man," in *History and Human Survival* (New York: Vintage, 1971). Here Lifton uses the word "formative" in the context of historical events.

8. Robert S. Wallerstein, "Psychoanalytic Perspectives on the Problem of Reality" (1973), in *Psychotherapy and Psychoanalysis* (New York: International Universities Press, 1975), 416–17.

9. Robert Waelder, "Psychoanalysis and History: Application of Psychoanalysis to Historiography," in *The Psychoanalytic Interpretation of History*, ed. Benjamin Wolman (New York: Harper, 1973), 3–30.

10. Jacques Barzun, *Clio and the Doctors* (Chicago: Chicago University Press, 1974), 14.

11. William Langer, "The Next Assignment" (Presidential Address to the American Historical Society), in *Psychoanalysis and History*, ed. B. Mazlish (New York: Grosset and Dunlap, 1971), 94–95.

12. Henry Krystal, "Trauma and the Stimulus Barrier," *Psychoanalytic Inquiry* 5 (1985): 135–62.

13. John Cohen, "Trauma and Repression," *Psychoanalytic Inquiry* 5 (1985): 165–90; C. Rycroft, *A Critical Dictionary of Psychoanalysis* (Totowa, N.J.: Littlefield, Adams, 1968), 171.

14. Terrence Des Pres, *The Survivor* (New York: Oxford University Press, 1976); Ilse Grubrich-Simitis, "Concretism to Metaphor: Children of Holocaust Survivors," in *The Psychoanalytic Study of the Child*, 53 vols. (New Haven, Conn.: Yale University Press, 1984), 39:301–19.

15. Maria Bergmann, "Thoughts on the Superego Pathology in Survivors and

Their Children," in *Generations of the Holocaust*, ed. Martin S. Bergmann and Milton E. Jucovy (New York: Basic Books, 1982), 263.

16. G. Minkowski, *"L'Anesthesie Affective,"* *Annales Medicales Psychologiques* (1946): 104, described *l'anesthesie affective*, that is, emotional insensitivity. Robert J. Lifton, "On Survivors," *History and Human Survival* (New York: Vintage, 1971), made the phrase the centerpiece of his work, tracing its origin to Freud, who described an "anesthetization of consciousness," which modern life requires to defend against modern horror.

17. American Psychiatric Association, *Diagnostic and Statistical Manual of Mental Disorders*, 4th ed. (Washington, D.C.: The American Psychiatric Association, 1994), 427.

18. Lifton, "On Survivors," 1970.

19. Martin Wangh, personal communication, 1982.

20. Dan Bar-On, "First Encounters Between Children of Survivors and Children of Perpetrators of the Holocaust," *Journal of Humanistic Psychology* 3364, (1993): 6–14. See also, Florence Kaslow, "Descendants of Holocaust Victims and Perpetrators: Legacies and Dialogue," *The International Connection* 9, no. 1 (1996): 12–23.

21. Anna Ornstein, "Survival and Recovery," *Psychoanalytic Inquiry* 5 (1985): 99–130.

22. Judith S. Kestenberg and Ira Brenner, "Le Narcissisme au Service de la Survie (Narcissism in the service of survival), *Revue Francaise de Psychoanalyse* 6 (1988): 1393–1408.

23. Paul Matussek, *Internment in Concentration Camps and Its Consequences* (1971; New York: Springer Verlag, 1975); Hillel Klein, presentation at a meeting of the New York Psychoanalytic Society, 1981.

24. Des Pres, *The Survivor*.

25. Hillel Klein, presentation at the New York Psychoanalytic Society, 1981.

26. Sylvia Axelrod, Ophilia Schnippper, and John Rau, "Hospitalized Offspring of Holocaust Survivors," *Bulletin of the Menninger Clinic* 44 (1980): 1–14.

27. Martin S. Bergmann and Milton E. Jucovy, eds., *Generations of the Holocaust* (New York: Basic Books, 1982).

28. Ornstein, "Survival and Recovery."

29. Judith S. Kestenberg, personal communication, 1992.

30. Judith S. Kestenberg "Survivor-Parents and Their Children" in *Generations of the Holocaust*, ed. Martin S. Bergmann and Milton E. Jucovy (New York: Basic Books, 1982), posits a universal "survivor complex."

31. Henry Krystal, ed., *Massive Psychic Trauma* (New York: International Universities Press, 1968).

32. Ornstein, "Survival and Recovery."

33. Kestenberg and Kestenberg, "The Experience of Survivor Parents."

34. William G. Niederland, "The Problem of the Survivor," *Journal of the Hillside Hospital* 10 (1961): 233–47.

35. Dorothy Rabinowitz, *New Lives* (New York: Alfred A. Knopf, 1976).

36. Maria Bergmann, "Thoughts on the Superego Pathology of Survivors and Their Children."

37. Robert Prince, *The Legacy of the Holocaust* (Ann Arbor, Mich.: UMI Research Press, 1985).

38. Judith S. Kestenberg, "Transposition Revisited: Clinical, Therapeutic, and Developmental Considerations," in *Healing Their Wounds: Psychotherapy with Holocaust Survivors and Their Families*, ed. Paul Marcus and Alan Rosenberg (New York: Praeger, 1989), 67–82.

3

Adult Survivors, Child Survivors, and Children of Survivors*

Judith S. Kestenberg

Differentiating the Holocaust from Other Trauma

It has been said that the Holocaust trauma resembles many other acute and chronic stress syndromes. One family therapist writing about the genocide committed on Jews, spoke of marital problems as "personal Holocausts."[1] Antiabortionists referred to abortion as a Holocaust because it kills unborn babies. Experts like Niederland spoke of a survivor syndrome and Eitinger of a concentration-camp syndrome.[2] Krystal applied the currently popular diagnosis, massive psychic trauma, to categorize the effect of the Holocaust. In my own view, the persecution of people in the Nazi era encompasses acute, chronic and recurrent, varying, successive, or simultaneous traumatizations, all of which are persecutory attacks upon the body and psyche of the victims.[3] Taken separately, each trauma also can be seen in traumatic stress disorders. Separation and losses can occur in other circumstances, as does illness, starvation, torture, and unjust imprisonment.

What is unique about the experience during the Holocaust? It was a government sanctioned and organized persecution of people who had no chance for redemption. Every victim of the Holocaust was persecuted; even those who escaped incarceration were in constant fear of being detected. For children of survivors, the fact that their parents had been persecuted is the single most important factor in their lives.

Life During the Holocaust

It must be acknowledged that during the Holocaust, adults and children were hounded by many—by government henchmen to be sure, but also by

---

*Originally presented as "The Holocaust: A Paradigm for Persecution" on May 11, 1991, at the American Psychiatric Meeting, New Orleans, LA.

neighbors, former friends, strangers, and extortionists. Each person, even a Jew, could be a potential source of danger in one's life. A chronic kind of emergency alarm had to function incessantly. One had to be vigilant and prepared for the worst. One had to be imaginative to get out of a trap. Each time, each day one survived was a miracle, an achievement. The persecutors cunningly tried to gain one's confidence, promising good conditions and leading the gullible to their deaths. In this process, the victims were humiliated and shamed in front of their friends and their children. Many were forced to become accomplices of their persecutors and to assume their guilt. Before they killed their victims, the Nazis did their utmost to corrupt them and prove their evil nature. Survival not only meant escaping death but keeping one's dignity and one's morality as a human being.[4]

The persecution was all-encompassing. It affected the victims' bodies until they became living skeletons. It destroyed the victims' sense of reality by creating an inferno, which could not be anticipated. It debased them, rendered them helpless and transformed many into hungry, wild animals who stepped on each other and fought for a piece of bread. The persecutors paraded before them, displaying their own strength, their cleanliness and elegance, looking down on the dirty, lowly creatures, the Jews. Of course the Jews were dirty and helpless because the Nazis made them so. By using pseudoeducational methods, the persecutors taught the persecuted to cower in fear, to use the toilet at specified times, and to be regulated in every other activity. Thus, they reduced the victims to the status of regimented infants. They brainwashed them not to believe in their own worth and to look up to the rulers as if they were gods. By hiding, many people—especially children—escaped the terror of the camps. But there was hiding in camps, too— in holes in the ground and by working on farms. Even when people were hidden in homes or convents, the constant fear of discovery and fear of displeasing the rescuer marked the hiding experiences as a precarious and uncertain haven from persecution.

This account has by no means exhausted the types of persecution to which the survivors were subjected. Can we expect, then, as Krystal does, that through self-healing and learning to mourn, survivors can integrate their past into the present and "accept the trauma as necessary?"[5] Can that be done? Is it possible to accept the Holocaust? Is it healthy to do it?

Coping with the Reality

The Holocaust was real. It is not a nightmare, not a bout of insanity.[6] It really happened. We must carefully study the means by which sane people could adjust and endure an insane world. Most important, we must learn to understand their endeavor to face the multiform experiences and study the means by which they, the persecuted return to a sane world and accept the new conditions.

However, we must also keep in mind that new conditions created a new form of persecution. Some returned to their homes and found no relatives but heard from their neighbors, "How come you are alive, Jankel?" They had no place to live, and their property had been taken. The Jewish community was decimated. Seeing the result of the persecution constituted a renewal of the experience of persecution. Their rescuers and the allied nations did not want to let them in and kept them in displaced persons' camps for years. In addition, when the survivors did reach the new countries, they were not greeted with enthusiasm. People did not believe their stories and did not want to listen to them. Even in Israel, people asked, "Why didn't you defend yourself?" They went through hell, and only the people who had been there with them could understand.

In the psychological treatment of trauma survivors, we, as therapists, have to descend into that hell and get to know it the best we can. Beyond our own nightmares and our own guilt feelings, which may find their way into the treatment room, listening daily to patients' accounts of trauma traumatizes the therapist, as well. Therapists, too, feel persecuted by the material.[7] The most difficult aspect of such treatment is the shared mourning in which the therapists must engage without losing track of their role as healers.

The elderly recount their losses and frequently have endured new losses, such as the death of a spouse, a brother, or sister. They are afraid to be alone. The new trauma is experienced once more as a persecution. "Why does this have to happen to me?" they ask. "Have I not suffered enough?"

It is very helpful for survivors to meet as a group. Once they have been together for a while and achieved a sense of trust, reminiscing allows the survivors to work through some of their persecutory anxiety by sharing it. In Sweden and in Los Angeles, Hedi Fried and Florabel Kinsler, respectively, have organized coffee houses for the aging survivors.[8] They meet, they eat, they talk, and they receive support from the staff. Others who need nursing care would be much better off in nursing homes for survivors. Being together with their fellow survivors creates a feeling for many that they have a family again or at least a community where they can feel understood. However, when they are alone and not in groups, they experience guilt. They know how it must have felt for their own parents to be left behind in Germany or to be separated upon arrival in Auschwitz to be sent to the gas chambers by themselves. Many younger adult survivors had to chose whether to stay with their parents or run away with their children. Whatever their decision, they feel guilty about it. They need an absolution of guilt so that they do not feel they deserve to die alone, unattended, and without a grave, as their parents did. Dr. Gertrud Hardtmann, a German psychoanalyst, made it her mission to visit the Jewish people in the old age home in Berlin. She tried to bring them solace and listen to them, but it took her a long time to gain their confidence and not to be seen as an enemy.

One elderly survivor, sick and alone, was able to reunite with two of his children in the United States. In his room, he erected a monument for his wife who had been gassed in Treblinka. His daughter, who survived, blamed him for his wife's death. He knew rationally it was not his fault, but his behavior indicated that he also punished himself for her death.

Speaking to Children

The question is asked over and over again: "Why can't the survivor talk to his children about his persecution?" Many need silence to work through their reminiscences in seclusion. Many are able to talk only to fellow survivors. Some of the parents whose children have been psychoanalyzed and whom we studied used their Holocaust experiences as threatening educational measures such as telling their children, "You don't want to eat and I had to eat mice, I was so hungry" or "Hitler did not kill me, but you will!"[9]

The survivors themselves want to leave their stories to their children and grandchildren, but they cannot bring themselves to tell their complete stories to the children directly. I believe that this is due to the fact that the children are looked upon as reincarnations of dead parents and relatives who will reproach them for their sins.

Survivors frequently want to shield their children or harden them against a future persecution. One survivor who had lost a wife and child in a ghetto of Romania concealed this fact from the family. Without talking about it, he selected his oldest child born after the war as a successor of his deceased child. He prepared her for starvation, lack of toilet facilities, and succeeded in getting her to ignore signals for hunger and elimination. She became emaciated, could not eat or go to the bathroom. She immersed herself in the Holocaust as if she lived in it. She transposed herself into her father's past and faithfully played the role of his deceased child, feeling more dead than alive. She had to revive this child for her father and had to perform brilliantly in place of the lost child.

CHILDREN OF SURVIVORS

Children who survived the Holocaust (with their parents or alone) are referred to as child survivors. When we speak of children of survivors, we refer to children born after the war.

Numerous interviews with children of survivors reveal that many feel they have a mission entrusted to them, to undo the Holocaust, to restore the parents' losses, to live out the aborted lives of the deceased, somehow to change history. This transposition onto the past, in which the messianic mission has to be fulfilled, prevents mourning. It is an attempt to restore the lost without mourning and to avoid facing the reality of the losses. There are numerous ways in which children of survivors fulfill their mission, or they may refuse: They may resent being chosen as rescuers and may turn away from the Holocaust in a phase of denial. Sometimes it is the parents who do not allow their children to play an important role in their rehabilitation. Instead, they shift the blame onto the child.[10] In any of these roles—rescuer, restorer, scapegoat—the children of survivors resemble those in dysfunctional families who have become the family delegates, performing functions and carrying out assigned missions, not necessarily in the best interest of their personal development.[11]

The Impossibility of Undoing the Holocaust

In one such family, the father berated his daughter continuously because she did not measure up to his three year old who died in the Holocaust. He did not feel comfortable in his role as a father of a new child, born after the war. He woke up this new child at night, and continuing his nightmare in her room, he attacked her as if she were a Nazi. Her very presence reminded him of his cardinal sin that he could not save his first little girl. The psychoanalysis of the daughter helped her to find a new identity. She gave up her role as an outcast, unworthy of life. She joined a cult that assured her acceptance everywhere in the country. She resumed her education and forgave her parents for mistreating her. She now became a help to them and allowed them to bask in her success. She was no longer afraid of her father, but in a reversal, assumed a maternal role toward him. The cult taught her to commune with the dead, permitting her to descend into her parents' past and understand them. When she came home, she was ready to achieve in the here and now and earn her parents' acceptance as a reward. Though it may require professional help, children of survivors can learn to relinquish their mission of undoing the Holocaust and restoring the dead to their parents. Only then can they help their parents to mourn and accept their losses.

CHILD SURVIVORS

When child survivors survive with their parents, they are frequently excluded from discussing the parents' or their own stories. Parents have a continuous need to protect their persecuted children from the effect of the persecution. Many capitalize on the common belief that children have not been traumatized because they did not understand what happened and cannot remember as their parents do. This parental attitude acts as a command to the child survivors not to remember and not to understand. In our interviews, child survivors frequently refer to themselves as having been too little to understand or remember. Sometimes it turns out that they were twelve to fourteen at the time and yet, like their parents, they perceive themselves as having been small children. In one instance, a child survivor who was eight years old when the persecution started told me that she could not remember anything and would have to ask her mother to answer the questions I put to her. Soon she began to spill her memories in a rapid succession. Then she stopped, terrified. She had not realized she could remember so much, and this insight produced a panic attack. We had to interrupt the interview and postpone it. Despite her best intentions to come back, she could never resume the interview.

In another instance, a child survivor approached me to help her remember an episode in her life that could not be recovered despite repeated attempts at hypnosis. It was not difficult to obtain this information from her by patiently asking for details.[12] Yet, when we reached the peak of the story, she suddenly reversed herself and said that she did not have to remember anything, and she stopped talking about it.

Memories of persecution and traumatization are repressed, denied, or disconnected from affect and from their deepest meaning. Child survivors, like their elders, still live in the Holocaust, yet most of them are quite capable of using their old survival strategies to adjust to their new lives. They have had an opportunity to study, learn a trade or profession, found a family, pursue a career, and achieve important goals in life. Many are in the helping professions while quite a few are artists and poets. In contrast to their parents, who often could not re-establish their careers and became depressed and defeated in their endeavor to achieve new important positions in exile, children took advantage of their opportunities. Progressive developmental forces helped the child survivors not only to survive but also to readjust. Unlike their parents, who kept their European identity, child survivors wanted to be "like everyone else," not different. They blended with their environment and sometimes did not let their friends know that they had been persecuted. They kept their nightmares to themselves and tried hard not to burden their children. Yet, they felt they had lost their childhood. When their children reached the age they had been at the time of persecution, they began to expect the worst for them. They could not play with their children.

If their parents had survived, child survivors frequently ended up being angry at them. They blamed their parents for abandoning them, giving them away into hiding, or separating from them in camps. They were ashamed of the parents' European manners, their accents, and their phobic behavior. At the other end of the spectrum, there were those who remained so attached to their mothers that they could not marry and have their own families. They remained forever children, protected by their parents and protecting them. When a parent died, these lonely people became depressed and felt even more isolated than before.

Most child survivors have a sense of not belonging anywhere. It was not unusual for them to have gone to school in one country and then have moved several times to other places, other countries, changing schools and languages, and being shunned everywhere by the native children. The memory of having been different from the non-Jewish Germans, Poles, or Czechs, who could go to school or to parks and could swim and play, looms large for these child survivors. Isolation from the community of other children was one of the most important deprivations of their lives.

Many of these children had to hide in order to survive. Some were even hidden in concentration camps. One was put in a pail to avoid detection by the SS guards. Another child who stood in line for the gas chamber with others in Auschwitz was grabbed by a woman and hidden under her skirt. We have records of two children who were hidden among corpses and one who hid herself among them. Her poem eloquently describes her feelings.

Recurrent Nightmare
Some nights
transport me back
to a time where absolute fear
was mine.

Like a stone between
dead bodies
I lie
holding my breath
afraid I'll die.

The earth
a cold wet
gritty slime
stiff limbs with
mine intertwine.

A shiver or twitch
will
reveal
that I am one
who still can feel.

I wait
with a pounding
heart
will the bullets
split
it apart?

I shut my eyes
so they won't see
the sadness, fear
inside
of me.

Irene Hizme

HEALING

Psychotherapeutic Interventions

In treating child survivors, we must be cognizant of their vulnerability to anything that might look to them as abandonment or discrimination. In their attempt to master their fear, they threaten the therapist with abandonment. They berate the therapist in transference and frequently mix up the persecutor with a parent or the therapist.[13] Though it is not logical, and though they may not be aware of it, child survivors hold their parents responsible for the persecutions they experienced. The situation becomes much more complicated for orphans. They tend to idealize their deceased parents and have severe loyalty conflicts, having to chose between the dead parents and the adoptive parents or foster parents. They are afraid to express their resentment against the dead who left them. This unexpressed aggression may engender depression and self-destructive acting out. Unbeknownst to the social workers of the 1940s and 1950s, these rescued orphans were better off in institutions, where they could be together and find friends, than they were in foster homes. The new friendships were valued, and separation from these friends was extremely painful. If one parent was still alive, jealousies arose to interfere with the friendship.

After the war, some child survivors who had been in orphanages or foster homes felt free to tell their stories. But after a while, they realized that people did not want to listen to them, that their stories branded them as different, and they became silent. Sometimes, we interview people who never knew another child survivor. Sometimes, when they were interviewed, as late as fifty years after the persecution ended, they felt a staggering relief at being able to unburden themselves.

Survivors also profit from participation in groups. A small percentage of child survivors needed treatment for depression, anxiety attacks, and problems with relationships to people. Anhedonia (absence of pleasure) is prevalent among young child survivors who were infants during the persecution. Alexithymia is an infrequent manifestation; however, certain of its features, such as not understanding and ignoring the signals of affects, are common. Sleep disturbances and somatic complaints are rarely reasons for seeking treatment, but are discovered when such patients come for treatment for other reasons.

Self-Healing

The self-healing process is much more pronounced in child survivors than in adult survivors. Though the child survivors are more likely to seek and achieve external success, the effects of having being persecuted and deprived still linger beneath the surface. Their self-healing is concentrated on being the same as the host population, blending in with the new environment and confiding only in fellow survivors.

Some adult survivors find solace by remembering and honoring their dead. They help to build monuments, collect oral histories, and generally commemorate the Holocaust. Creativity is one of the self-healing processes that yields cultural products, such as paintings or poetry, that can be shared with the community. Individual altruistic attitudes are characteristic. No child could survive who was not helped by an adult. The identification with the rescuer leads to altruism.

If one can put the differences succinctly, if not precisely, one can say that adult survivors tend to be either depressed and defeated or overachievers, overly successful in compensation for the experienced depreciation. Children of survivors, born after the war, tend to enter a time tunnel that brings them back to their parents' Holocaust experience, where they hope to retrieve the dead. Once they return to the present reality, they learn to help their parents mourn their losses.

Child survivors mourn their lost childhood and their lost parents, and try to mend by becoming like the others who were not persecuted. Children of survivors also try to make themselves indistinguishable from their surroundings. When they accept themselves as survivors, as Europeans, as Jews, they become capable of sharing with one another and mourning together.

In confronting the Holocaust trauma and its sequelae, ultimately one has to admit, in Paul Zeslis' words, "I try to understand, to at least comprehend the past—the Holocaust. Still I cannot, I cannot. I am left staring out over the abyss, into the void."[14]

NOTES

1. Israel W. Charny in collaboration with Chanan Rapaport, *How Can We Commit the Unthinkable? Genocide: The Human Cancer* (Boulder, Colo.: Westview Press, 1981).

2. William G. Niederland, "The Problem of the Survivor," *Journal of the Hillside Hospital* 10 (1961): 233–47; L. Eitinger, "Jewish Concentration Camp Survivors," in *The Holocaust and Its Perseverance*, ed. O. Ayalon and L. Eitinger et al. (Assen, The Netherlands: Van Gorcum, 1983).

3. Henry Krystal, ed., *Massive Psychic Trauma* (New York: International Universities Press, 1968); Henry Krystal, *Integration and Self-Healing* (Hillsdale, N.J.: The Analytic Press, Lawrence Erlbaum Assoc. Inc., 1988).

4. Jean Amery, *At the Minds Limits* (New York: Schocken Books, 1977); Primo Levi, *Survival In Auschwitz* (New York: Collier Books, 1959).

5. Krystal, *Integration*.

6. Ilse Grubrich-Simitis, "Extreme Traumatization as Cumulative Trauma," in

The Psychoanalytic Study of the Child, 53 vols. (New Haven, Conn.: Yale University Press, 1981), 36:415–50.

7. Yael Danieli, "Countertransference in the Treatment and Study of Nazi Holocaust Survivors and Their Children," *Victimology: An International Journal* 5 (1981): 3–4.

8. See chapter 14, this volume.

9. Eva Fogelman, "Intergenerational Group Therapy: Child Survivors of the Holocaust and Offsprings of Survivors," *Psychoanalytic Review* 75, no. 4 (1988): 619–40.

10. Ibid.

11. Helm Stierlin, *Psychoanalysis and Family Therapy* (New York: Jason Aronson, 1977).

12. Judith S. Kestenberg, "Memories from Early Childhood," *Psychoanalytic Review* 75, no. 4 (1988): 561–71.

13. Transference occurs during psychotherapy when the patient directs to the therapist some feelings and thoughts originating elsewhere in relation to others.

14. Paul D. Zislis, "Creative Writing: The Witness," *Jefferson Journal of Psychiatry* 5 (1987): 83–86.

4

Man Behind Walls

Kazimierz Godorowski

Man always lives to some extent behind the walls of his defenses. But most men do not have to lead an existence behind the walls of ghettos and concentration camps where the familiar personal defenses become virtually irrelevant.

This chapter describes the situations of maximum stress created by the Germans in occupied Polish territories during World War II, and examines some attitudinal, behavioral, and personality changes fomented by the conditions of life imposed upon ghetto inmates.

An analysis of *Mein Kampf* and public speeches by Hitler and his associates, beginning in 1920, as well as the German internal and foreign policy throughout the entire period of Nazism, reveals that their superordinate idea was antisemitism. Indeed, Jozef Wolff believed that the main aim of the aggression against Poland was the annihilation of Jews. Wolfgang de Boor, in his biography of Hitler, writes explicitly that the "[m]ilitary activities, and particularly starting the war in the East, were designed to serve the far reaching goal of annihilation of Jews as well as decimation of Slavic nations who lived in the German-occupied territories of Europe."[1]

Kogon subsumes ghettos under the category of concentration camps.[2] Enumerating Third Reich concentration camps, he includes ghettos in Warsaw, Lodz, Lwow, and Ryga because ghettos served as a repository for the "racially unwanted element" of the Third Reich and the occupied territories until the "Final Solution" was implemented. The ghettos enabled the Germans to keep this mass of people under their strict control, employing a relatively small police force and conserving their material resources and physical strength for military purposes and warfare production. In the ghettos, the Jews were isolated under the worst possible living conditions. The Jewish population was "slandered, humiliated, broken and annihilated."[3] Purposely creating a system of extreme-stress situations made ghetto administration easier and made the inhabitants' daily existence most difficult materially and psychologically.

Stress, as it is understood in psychological science, can be defined as "all outside factors, which make it more difficult or impossible to fulfill one's needs and to perform one's planned activities; create danger or influence one's personality in such a way that one's self-esteem is lowered."[4] Extremely stressful situations can result either from unforeseen occurrences, such as natural disasters—catastrophic floods, earthquakes, volcanic eruptions—or from planned human activities, such as the deliberate extermination of the Jewish people. During the Nazi regime in the Third Reich, not only Jews, but Gypsies, were victims of such a deliberate, stress-inducing policy; all Slavic nations were to experience it in the totalitarian systems that followed. As a result of ideology, certain groups of people were arbitrarily defined as less valuable, or simply harmful, according to racial and class criteria, and were sentenced to rejection, contempt, deportation, or physical annihilation.

Extreme conditions were deliberately created in the ghettos and concentration camps.[5] Hunger and fear were the dominating conditions, and the external situation on the war front prevented any possibility of defense. Fulfillment of biological and psychological needs was also made impossible, as well as the performance of planned tasks and life plans. Thus, everyday life in a ghetto comprised all the situations that create stress.

A campaign to make a nation detestable was in progress. The constant prospect of perishing in one of the camps, and especially the impotence in the face of these conditions, created almost intolerable emotional tensions, rendered previously useful mechanisms of defense irrelevant, and often led to disorganization of behavior.

The prevailing conditions in these totalitarian settings included: forced separation from the society in which one used to live; assignment to a specific group (in sets of contrasting groups of people, such as jailers and prisoners); the necessity to establish a certain social position in the group; forced compliance with the rules governing virtually all aspects of life; forced adaptation to values totally at variance with those that were functional in the world at large; and deprivation of freedom of movement, including the impossibility of leaving and the loss of hope of ever being able to leave. All the above-mentioned factors and the attendant feelings of isolation and separation from one's social group, the awareness of constant threat, and the sense of hopelessness and helplessness constituted mainly psychological stresses.

In addition, there was constant hunger and an unbelievable population density. This intensified after the liquidation of the small-town ghettos and the deportation of their inhabitants to larger ones. The intensified population density, in turn, increased the ever-present hunger.

In the ghettos, the mass occurrence of biological emaciation ending in death by starvation induced a so-called "corrosion of personality structure," and changed the inmates' hierarchy of needs and values. In the end, their will to oppose was broken and was substituted by total psychic obedience toward authority. Through these measures, the Germans succeeded in increasing their control over masses of people. It was clearly recognized that permanent hunger can determine human behavior and psychological attitudes, as well as personality changes. The symptoms and effects of starvation were described by Jewish physicians in the ghettos and physicians working in the concentration camps.[6] According to the testimony of ghetto, concentration camp, and death camp survivors, hunger was the dominant problem.[7] It was not by accident that Nazi authorities rationed food to an absolute minimum level in the ghettos and camps. Their purpose was not to economize to support the war, but to deprive and dehumanize the ghetto and camp inhabitants.

A permanently hungry person became vulnerable to any manipulations; psychologically weak personalities were tempted into collaboration. A ghetto inhabitant had to focus all his efforts on getting even a little bit of food for himself and his family.[8] Hunger changed the hierarchy of needs and values and pushed the instinct for self-survival onto an even higher plane. One of the truly devilish ideas was the offer (during one of the "actions" [*Aktion*] in the Warsaw ghetto in 1942) of a loaf of bread as a lure to induce the ghetto inmates to come voluntarily to the *Umschlagplatz* (place of assembly). It was an event without precedent in the Warsaw ghetto, and despite efforts by the Opposition Movement to counteract it, it greatly contributed to the ease of carrying out one more Nazi "action," such as rounding up the Jews for slave labor or for transport to extermination camps.

From a somatic point of view, the main symptom of hunger is rapid and great weight loss. A wide range of psychic changes also occur that influence the total personality. The psychopathological changes appear in three phases: The first phase resembles neurasthenia, and its characteristic feature is a food complex, insofar as food has taken on a specific extra value and thoughts about food dominate a person's consciousness. In the second phase, deliria and dream states occur with partial or full amnesia, hallucinations, and delusions. Moral restraints crumble at the prospect of getting a piece of bread, even at the expense of one's closest relatives. Finally, in the third phase, apathy, a reluctance to exert any kind of effort, and indifference toward the environment set in. A protracted condition of undernourishment leads to irreversible somatic and psychic changes resembling the last stage of the so-called crisis of identity. In the camps, this condition was given the name *musselmann*.[9] It is the final effect of a multifaceted biological and psychical deprivation.

In analyses of the ghetto, this phenomenon is too rarely considered a factor contributing to the population's apparent passivity and lack of will to resist. In fact, this outcome was unavoidable after many months or even years of severe biological and physical stress. Toward the end, most of the inmates were unable to perform either mental or physical work and, except for a few, yielded passively to their fate.

Though the contents of *Mein Kampf*—published long before the outbreak of World War II and translated into many languages—did not leave any doubts as to the fate of Jews in the Third Reich (and consequently in the occupied territories), even the greatest pessimists were unable to foresee the *Endlösung* (or "Final Solution," that is, extermination). It was incomprehensible.

Deportation, either from the native country or from a small town to a main ghetto, constituted the first step in separation from the familiar background. The subsequent economic ruin and the complete social degradation were felt especially keenly by the intelligentsia, or the free professionals.[10] German Jews harbored the greatest illusions—and suffered the gravest disillusionment. A large part of the German-Jewish population had assimilated, contributing enormously to the artistic, economic, and cultural life of Germany. Many had even shed blood for Germany in World War I. Therefore, they felt their fate more deeply than the rest of European Jewry and could not fathom the *Endlösung*. In the United States, in 1940, nobody believed what was going on in the camps, even though conditions at that time were far from having reached rock-bottom. The same disbelief possessed Polish couriers who saw ghettos with their own eyes.[11] Simply put, Europeans and Americans at that time could not grasp the murder of a whole nation.[12]

The first step, then, was a general pauperization of European-Jewish society and the deprivation of the possibility of a normal existence.[13] Even after official announcements from the highest authorities in the Third Reich (which left no room for doubts about the plans for total annihilation), and notwithstanding deportation, isolation in the ghettos, and the creation of horrible living conditions, still the possibility of total annihilation was denied. A so called "make-believe life" was created. For example, it was believed that the war would end sooner than the annihilation and that the Nazi regime would ultimately decide against the *Endlösung*. After all, Europeans of that time, including Jews, were not programmed for such horror. It was indeed "the end of our world."[14]

Difficult situations must not be confused with extreme situations. Difficult situations constantly exist and may even be dramatic in effect. However, their elements fit into a set of norms and common experiences and do not exceed certain limits. We are basically "conditioned" for all such situations. But the Jewish experience during the Nazi regime was absolutely above and beyond any pre-existing cognitive scheme. Man lost his trust in man; he could find neither models for his attitudes and behavior, nor adequate and effective mechanisms to defend against a pervasive fear. In other words, familiar mechanisms of adaptation and existing values were rendered not

only meaningless, but proved actually destructive when applied to these extreme conditions.

Robbed of our defense systems based on defined ethical systems and rules
of social co-existence, we are at a loss to create new ones adequate to the moment. The ghetto and concentration camp conditions presented a completely
alien juxtaposition of the individual to the surrounding world, necessitating a
new hierarchy of values at odds with the old cognitive structures. Under such
stress, it is impossible to create defense mechanisms necessary for maintaining
individual and group identity and a stable psychic balance.

Till the last moment, Jews in Poland did not believe that they would be
totally annihilated.[15] Such conviction constituted denial, one of the most
comprehensible mechanisms of defense. In the service of that denial, inhabitants did not believe reports from death camp runaways. I, personally, remember being told the story of a Treblinka runaway while I was working
with a group of Jews in one of the German firms in Bialystok. The Jews
treated the story as *Greuelpropaganda* (horror stories), and some even spec-
ulated that it was propaganda by the leaders of the Opposition Movement,
a self-defense organization. Instead of rallying behind the Opposition Movement, the general ghetto population gathered around the *Judenrat* (Jewish
governing council) in attempts to buy off the Germans with work, foreign
currency, and jewelry, hoping this would enable them to survive the war
and win the race with time.

Denial of total annihilation was especially evident among Western European Jews, who were sometimes even transported to death camps in open
trains. In contrast, the sober analysis of the situation in the ghetto, which
took the military-front situation into consideration, pointed at only minute
chances of survival. Whoever could tried at all costs to go to the so-called
"Aryan side" (beyond the confines of the ghettos) or to send children there,
but sometimes only one of many children could be saved, creating an unbearable moral dilemma. The emotional situation was worse for ghetto families than it was for death-camp inmates. The latter, ignorant of the fate of
their "free" relatives, believed that they would survive.

Yet, even getting to the "Aryan side" did not assure survival. The general
population was threatened with death for each and every case of helping Jews,
and this threat, compounded by dangerous blackmailers—the so-called
Shmalcovnics—discouraged otherwise willing people from aiding Jews.
Therefore, only a small group living outside ghettos helped to rescue Jews.

The occupying authorities fostered antisemitic attitudes through intensive
propaganda. For example, before each German "action" in the Bialystok
ghetto, the whole city was papered with a huge quantity of colorful hand-
bills, only just the size of a matchbox, with a picture of a louse representing
the head of a Jew with side locks and a skullcap. Similar huge posters were
hung all over the city. Big boards reading *"Achtung, Seuchengefahr"* ("Attention, danger of epidemic") were attached to ghetto gates. In fact, the

danger of epidemic in the Jewish ghetto was spawned by forced isolation, hunger, and deprivation of even the most elementary medical care.

Jewish resistance was weakened by this deprecating picture of themselves, which on some level caused them to feel responsible for the spread of lice and contagious diseases. Understandably, such conditions engendered a crisis of identity in a psychologically weakened people. The loss of their former conditions of life further threatened their identity, as it required a re-evaluation of needs and values; undermined identification with other members of the group; and generally produced deep personality changes.

For example, the Germans deluded the members of the *Judenrat* and the *Ordnungsdienst* (local Jewish police) into believing that they and their families would be spared the worst, a promise obviously not to be kept, but one that led some to collaborate. Thus, altruism and tolerance gave way to egoism at all cost—and the price was high indeed. Under stress, the "fight or flight" syndrome prevails. When neither fight nor flight is possible, as in the case of totalitarian institutions, the only recourse is to create new defense mechanisms, "specific reactions to psychic stresses," reactions that consist of applying spontaneous stress-reducing mechanisms to immutable stress situations.[16]

In the camps and ghettos, an often-used defense mechanism was the creation of a "psychic reservation," that is, an artificial "lifelike" situation, in an attempt to at least partially ignore the reality. This was a sort of psychic escape from the horror of life in "the city of the death."[17] Frankl called this defense mechanism the "armored layer," Kogon called it "protective armor plate," and Lepinski "camp autism."[18] Fantasizing while being awake was another defense mechanism. These defenses involve an apparent indifference toward one's surroundings, not out of callousness, but from actual helplessness and an inhibition of the impulses to avoid real danger. But the most frequently used defense mechanism, which might even be viewed as a form of auto-therapy, was the rejection of reality by means of denial.

As already mentioned, contemporary Europeans were simply not "programmed" for the possibility of destroying an entire nation.[19] Therefore, until the omnipresent and merciless hunger and its effects reduced individuals to the level of a mere vegetative state, Jews in the ghettos created a substitute life consisting of lecture series, research on the symptoms of hunger diseases, and the creation of art. Characteristically, this led to the desperate creation of hopeful illusions. The Latin saying *contra spem spero* (to hope against all [probability of] hope) is pertinent here. The ghetto population believed any piece of information indicating an increase of the chances to survive, to win the race with time for life. Since they paid more attention to local information than to news from the distant war fronts, their optimism was awakened by word that ghetto "shops" had received huge orders from the *Wehrmacht* or from German firms. Similarly, hope and unwarranted optimistic conclusions were drawn from careful observations of the personnel changes in the *Judenrat* and the local *Gestapo*.[20] An increase in religious and mystical feelings can also be understood as a defense mechanism. In the ghetto, as in Vilna, people embarked upon spiritual, even messianic missions.[21] From a psychological point of view, these were desperate attempts at psychical self-defense and therefore can be considered defense mechanisms.

Different attitudes developed among ghetto inhabitants, depending on their personality structure, level of psychic strength, and the current military situation. Attitudes became polarized. People became timid, bewildered, thoughtless, pessimistic, realistic, or broken.[22] Optimists yielded to illusions. Active, brutal, opportunistic individuals with a strong will cooperated with the apparatus of terror. Others were gullible. Whether one became resigned, prosocial, asocial, or antisocial greatly depended also on a person's maturity and individual hierarchy of attitudes and values.[23] These attitudes changed depending on external camp reality, hunger conditions, internal personality factors, and the situation on the war fronts.

An analysis and ethical evaluation of the Holocaust should take into account the Germans' system of "antipsychotherapy" and "antipedagogy."[24] Privileges were given to those who had been broken and who accepted asocial and antisocial attitudes. These people helped the Nazis carry out their extermination plans. Indeed, the excesses of the *Ordnungsdienst* in the ghettos and the *Kapos* (overseers) in the death camps even today evoke the feeling of horror. They exemplified the effectiveness of extreme negative stimulae in manipulating weak people.

In retrospect, not all members of the *Ordnungsdienst* and the *Kapos* can be considered clinical psychopaths, notwithstanding the fact that they often undertook the role of executioner (by selecting other people) in order to save their own lives. Like every other inmate, the *Kapos* were weak and had reached the point of identity crisis; for them survival at all cost was the only thing that mattered. Under normal conditions they might never have become criminals.

Postwar data point to the hypothesis that, for the Third Reich, ghettos were not only a source of slave labor, but also served as laboratories where mass-killing methods could be developed semisurreptitiously, without a manifest acknowledgment of engaging in racial genocide.[25] Even before the unspeakably terrifying Holocaust was decided upon, the ghetto inmates were killed *in extremis* by hunger, lack of medical care, constant fear, and dehumanization. Finally, the hope to survive failed and transformed into utter hopelessness.

NOTES

1. Wolfgang de Boor, *Hitler Mensch–Übermensch–Untermensch* (Hitler: Man, superman, subhuman) (Frankfurt am Main: R. G. Fischer, 1985).

2. Eugen Kogon, *Der SS-Staat: Das System der deutschen Konzentrationslager* (The SS state: The system of German concentration camps) (München: Verlag Karl Alber, 1974), 157.

3. Ibid., 34.

4. Andrzej Lewicki, *Psychologia Kliniczna* (Clinical psychology) (Warsaw: Wydawnictwa Uniwersytetu Adama Mickiewicza, 1969).

5. Bruno Bettelheim, *The Informed Heart: The Human Condition in Modern Mass Society* (New York: The Free Press, 1960).

6. Ludwig Hirszfeld, *Historia jednego zycia* (History of one life) (Warsaw: Czytelnik, 1946); Stanislaw Sterkowicz, ed., *Przeglad, Lekarski Osw* 1 (Remarks on concentration camp hunger emaciation) (Kracow: Zwigzek-Wydawnictwa Literackiego, 1971).

7. Kazimierz Godorowski, *Psychologia i psychopatologia hitlerowskich obozow koncentracyjnych* (Psychology and psychopathology of Nazi concentration camps) (Warsaw: Akademia Teologii Katolickiej, 1985).

8. Olga Wormser-Migot, *Le systeme concentrationnaire nazi 1933–1945* (The Nazi concentration camp system 1933–1945) (Paris: Presses Universitaries de France, 1968).

9. A Muslim (who accepts his fate)

10. Else Behrend-Rosenfeld and Georg Luckner, *Lebenszeichen aus Piaski* (Signs of life from Piaski) (München: Fischer, 1970).

11. Jan Nowak-Jezioranski and Jan Karski, *Kurier z Warszawy* (Krakow: Republica Instytut Wydawnictwa Znak, 1979).

12. Walter Laquer, *The Terrible Secret* (London: Weidenfeld and Nicolson, 1983).

13. Philip Friedman, *Roads to Extinction: Essays on the Holocaust* (Philadelphia: Jewish Publication Society of America, 1980).

14. Tadeusz Holuj, *Raj* (Paradise) (Warsaw: Czytelnik, 1974).

15. Tomasz Szarota, *Okupowanej Warszawy dzien powszedni* (Everyday life in occupied Warsaw) (Warsaw: Czytelnik, 1988).

16. Lewicki, *Clinical Psychology*, 59.

17. Hirszfeld, *History of One Life*.

18. Viktor Frankl, *Psycholog w obozie Koncentratcyjnym* (Psychologist in a concentration camp) (Warsaw: Wydawnictwo Literackie, 1962); Kogon, *The SS State*; Antoni Lepinski, *Rytm zycia* (Life rhythm) (Kracow: Wydawnictwo Literackie, 1972).

19. Frankl, *Psychologist*; E. Cohen, *"Reakcja poczatkowa na osadzenie w obozie koncentracyjnym"* (Initial reaction to confinement in concentration camp), *Przeglad, Lekarski Osw* 1, ed. Stanislaw Sterkowicz.

20. H. G. Adler, *Theresienstadt 1941–1945. Das Antlitz einer Zwanggemeinschaft* (Theresienstadt 1941–1945. The aspect of a compulsory society) (Tübingen: J. C. B. Mohr, 1955).

21. Friedman, *Roads to Extinction*.

22. Adler, *Theresienstadt*.

23. Henry Krystal, *Massive Psychic Trauma* (New York: International Universities Press, 1968).

24. Kazimierz Godorowski, "Antypsychoterapia i antypedagogika—wzorce totalitarnej socjotechniki, Przegl. Lek" (Antipsychotherapy and antipedagogy—models of totalitarian sociotechnic) *Medical Review* 43, no. 1 (1986): 17–20.

25. Kazimierz Godorowski, *Psychology and Psychopathology of Nazi Concentration Camps*; Andrea Devoto, *Il Comportamento Umano in Condizioni Estreme* (Human conditions in extreme situations) (Milan: Franco Angeli, 1985).

5

Interviewing for Indemnification*

Milton Kestenberg

After World War II, Holocaust survivors arriving in the United States or elsewhere often were very badly hurt, retraumatized by the disbelief of the communities where they settled. People did not believe that the atrocities described really happened; oftentimes they did not even want to listen. Many survivors were faced by the disbelief of their immediate families, the very ones who had facilitated their admission to the United States. A well-known example is the story of the child who told her American aunt how starved she had been, whereupon the aunt told her how hard it was during the war in the United States because sugar had been rationed. Survivors were accused of exaggeration, if not outright fabrication.

This chapter will inform you about the remedies available against the government of Germany for crimes and atrocities committed by the Nazis. First I shall list the conditions under which such remedies are available. Then I shall discuss the role of the physicians and what they can do to support the survivor's claim when the claim is based on physical or psychological aftereffects of the Holocaust experience.

The details of the procedure for indemnification is usually explained to the claimant by a lawyer or an agency. Many patients need much support and assistance in pursuing their claims to their best advantage because the conflicts pertaining to "blood money" from Germany are such that they lead to confusion, misunderstanding of what is required, forgetting, or misstatements of facts to the German-appointed physicians.

Under the German Indemnification Laws, a survivor whose earning capacity was reduced by at least 25 percent due to persecution is entitled to

*Presented in different form at the American Psychiatric Association Annual Meeting, 1991, New Orleans, LA.

a pension. At the beginning of the program, the medical experts, retained by the German government to examine the survivors who filed a claim, in many instances capriciously would recognize a disability of 24 percent or less and they recommend a rejection of the claim. As a rule, the physicians' recommendations were accepted by the indemnification authorities.

The procedure was very complex and before the claim was submitted to the medical experts in Germany, the claimant had to go through prolonged and rigorous red tape. The Supreme Court of Germany, the *Bundesgerichtshof*, ruled that in accordance with the provisions of the indemnification laws, a claimant may reopen his case if he can prove the exacerbation of his disability, that is, *Verschlimmerung*. Reconsideration of the original claim required a number of conditions to be met.[1]

An application for review for reasons of the exacerbation of the disability must be accompanied by a medical certificate. For this certificate to be acceptable, the physician must qualify according to stringent standards and submit a detailed report on the treatment of the patient.[2]

Once the patient's disability is recognized by the German authorities, the physician can recommend to the patient to apply for a course of treatment, a so-called *Heilverfahren*, which may include going to a health resort. The patient then would make periodic applications for reimbursement for medical expenses, such as physicians' fees, medicines, nursing care, and related expenses.

The reports prepared by the physician are submitted to the German indemnification offices and then forwarded to a physician appointed and trusted by the German government, a *Vertrauensarzt*, who maintains offices within the consular district of the claimant. These physicians are experts in their respective medical fields. They also examine the patient and submit appropriate reports to the German authorities, in German. They take into consideration the report of the treating physician. The German authority submits both reports to an expert at a German university for a final determination.

In the event of the patient's death, the physician should certify that there is a causal connection between the ailment, caused by the persecution, and the patient's death. An example of this might be a suicide due to posttraumatic depression. If the German consulate recognizes that such a causal relationship exists, the family is entitled to reimbursement for burial expenses. Furthermore, if a widow can establish, to the satisfaction of the German indemnification authorities, that a causal relationship exists between the ailment resulting from persecution for which a pension had been paid and the cause of death, a widow's pension will be paid. A widow's pension equals 60 percent of the pension collected by the deceased spouse.

With the advance of medical knowledge, the link between persecution and a subsequent disability or death was frequently recognized in the United States, but not necessarily by the German medical establishment. However, with the greater understanding of posttraumatic stress disorders (PTSD) during the course of the decades since the end of World War II, the German medical practice probably has changed, too. In any case, it is worthwhile to reopen a claim for an older survivor, especially since the granting of a pension to a survivor will also benefit his widow, who, without it, is frequently destitute. The pensions received from Germany, in addition to social security payments, enable aging survivors to spend the eve of their lives in dignity without resorting to public welfare and charity.

There were times when misguided German experts treated applications with prejudice. Now, since the program is at its conclusion, their attitudes have mellowed.[3] One must add that at the beginning of this program, when mental illnesses were not considered a cause for indemnification, German medicine adhered to outmoded psychiatric tenets. Since then, the German psychiatric literature has advanced considerably.[4]

During the years of my practice as an attorney, filing and processing German indemnification claims, I found that the granting or denial of a claim has great emotional impact on the survivor. A denial of the claim by Germany was, in a way, a disavowal of the survivor's veracity. Thus, the refusal was experienced as an attack on the survivor's human dignity, similar to the degradation suffered during the Holocaust and after, when the survivors' accounts of their experiences were greeted with disbelief. In effect, it was a continuation of the persecution.[5]

A client whose claim had been rejected came to my office, his shirt open, screaming, "Let them kill me!" I had great difficulty persuading him to file an appeal. In his excitement, he again screamed, "I don't want their money—I cannot face my children." Later, when he was informed that his appeal was granted, he came to my office with his entire family. We did not talk about money. "Do you know what saved me during the war?" he asked. "I promised my mother to protect my younger brother, Josele. We both survived, nobody else." It seemed as if, at last, the Germans had recognized his right to have survived.

I learned to ask pertinent questions or reassure the clients to facilitate the flow of information and to allow them to understand the connection between the present ailment and the past trauma. A simple example is a case of a woman who suffered from a knee injury whose source was unknown. Her request for compensation was refused because she could not find a link between her present handicap and the persecution. I helped her relax and asked her to tell me what had happened in her childhood in Germany. Her father had been taken away by the Gestapo. I asked her to describe the parting scene. She was present when the SS men came to arrest her father. She threw herself on him trying to prevent the intruders from taking him away, whereupon one of the Nazis kicked her in the leg and removed her. She had not forgotten the incident, but never connected it to her present condition. People say to us during our research interviews: "Now that you asked me, I recall. . . ."

The art of interviewing is to know what to ask. A woman afraid of monsters was amazed when I asked whether the monsters wore helmets. "How did you know that?" she asked, and promptly recollected seeing helmeted German soldiers killing civilians.[6][7]

Guilt feelings also prevent the traumatized survivors from remembering traumatic and even pretraumatic experiences. A woman who remembered parting from her mother (who had asked her to run away when she heard the Gestapo pounding on the door), could not remember the face of her mother at all. When I explained to her that she could have been shot running away while her mother had a chance to survive in a labor camp, she was relieved and suddenly remembered the color of her mother's hair and eyes. She had feared that recalling her mother's face would bring back all the good things her mother had done for her before the persecution and thus aggravate her guilt for abandoning her mother. When she was reassured, she could afford to remember. Incidents like this one, showing that present-day incapacitating feelings of guilt and depression can derive from the circumstances of persecution, are very convincing to the German authorities.

Sometimes people came to me after they had been examined by the *Vertrauensarzt*. These doctors were German-speaking immigrants. Some of them were compassionate people, but not all. One was exceptionally rigid. He followed a list of questions and did not allow the claimants to speak freely, demanding that they stick to the topic. The whole interview impressed my clients as a hostile interrogation and brought back to their minds the brutality of the Gestapo or of the doctors in concentration camps. The survivors regressed, had renewed nightmares, and suffered from severe anxiety. Interviewing them in my office to elicit information that would be helpful to them required listening first to what the examining doctor had said to them and how they had reacted. In one instance, I was able to submit my lengthy interview to the *Vertrauensarzt*, who then changed his mind and gave a favorable report.

A significant number of clients thought there was nothing wrong with them. They believed they must feign sickness in order to outsmart the Germans and to get a pension. They sometimes asked me what to say to the examining physician in order to appear sick. My advice that they tell the truth was not always acceptable because it branded them as sick—which they denied to themselves. I had to elicit information that they could truthfully share with the doctor, such as sleeplessness, nightmares, phobic behavior, and a bad temper—symptoms suffered by many elderly survivors who had been hit on the head repeatedly or who had contracted encephalitis.

It was very important to realize that many survivors held on to their symptomatic self-healing methods and refused help. For instance, when I directed those with nightmares to a sleep laboratory where they could receive medication, they would arrange to go on a vacation. One of them had an accident, broke a bone, and could not come to his appointment.[8]

Quite a few were afraid to come to my office by themselves. They had to be accompanied by their spouses or their children, who acted as spokespersons. They did not recognize their anxiety and their phobic need for a protector. In fact, many of their symptoms were camouflaged by such excuses as not being able to speak English well, not ever having ventured further than their immediate neighborhood, or fearing they might get lost. At the same time, they did not want their children to know the full extent of their shame and could not say much in front of them.

Some people who had been granted indemnities had moved away and did not report to my office to collect their monies, which I hold in trust. Notoriously, adult survivors would not make claims on behalf of their children, whom they wanted to protect. In many ways, they pretended to themselves that the children had not been traumatized. They wanted to spare them the persecutory interrogation they themselves had experienced.

In the reports it is important to present the history of the patient chronologically and then connect the traumatizing events with the present symptoms and exacerbations of symptoms. The patients are often unable to organize their story in a comprehensive fashion. The clearer the picture is to the examining physician and the German professional expert, the less doubt it arouses in their minds about whether the claim is justified. It is also important to show that before the persecution the patient functioned adequately, so that it cannot be said that his ailment is constitutional or stems from before the persecution.

The re-examination for exacerbation claims is dreaded by the survivor. He is justly afraid that he will have a more significant relapse than he already has had. This is hardly ever taken into consideration by the examining physician. Until relatively recently, people who had suffered great hardships and had never applied for compensation could bring their claims to the Jewish Claim Commission. What they could receive was the grand sum of $2,500. The commission had to follow the rules imposed by the German government. For that reason, the application process did not lose its original persecutory quality, although it was reduced by the fact that the claimant went to a Jewish-staffed office.

There are still many survivors whose claims have been rejected or who could but would not apply for compensation, who would like to do so now. In the beginning, when psychiatric claims by adults were accepted, many of the claims by child-victims were not accepted because the Germans reasoned that they could not have been traumatized since they could not remember the trauma. It is not too late to reopen these claims. When the law was changed, the previously rejected claimants were not notified. Many did not know that they could now apply for treatment of depressions or anxiety states and for mental hospital stays. It is not too late to reopen these claims.

There are child survivors who were too young to be able to apply for themselves earlier on, and now that they are adults, would like to have their claims heard. In October 1989, at a workshop under the leadership of Professor Kisker at the University of Hanover, compensation—not only for Jews, but for Gypsies and for Germans who had been sterilized—was discussed. As a member of the workshop, I helped draft a petition to the German government requesting reconsideration of these previously rejected, or previously not legalized claims, and extension of the deadline for submitting applications.[9]

Clearly, it is important for a treating or consulting psychiatrist to be acquainted with the existing laws and with the obstacles that stand in the way of the claimants. Similarly, I have tried to show that sensitive interviewing techniques on the part of a consulting lawyer can overcome psychological obstacles to remembering, the fear of the authorities, and the reluctance and shame connected with requesting "blood money." Lawyers as well as physicians and psychiatrists can elicit the information that will help a survivor obtain a pension, or an increase in the present pension, under the existing law.

NOTES

1. (a) That the original application was filed prior to December 31, 1969; (b) That the medical examiner recognizes the increase in the claimant's disability by at least 20 percent, and 30 percent for claimants over the age of 68; (c) That the claimant's disability had been recognized in the original decision, but only to the extent of less than 25 percent; (d) That the original decision was favorable to the claimant and afforded him a pension, which was subsequently canceled on the grounds that on reexamination the claimant's health was improved; and (e) That certain symptoms related to persecution were listed in the original application but ignored in the reports of the medical experts on which the decision was made; and that these symptoms have a bearing on the present exacerbation.

2. This certificate has to contain information as to the professional standing of the physician, such as membership in professional societies, teaching positions, or a board-certified specialty, and a list of publications related to the ailment causing the disability. The physician should provide all the dates of consultation or treatment based on his records and a list of medicines prescribed; instances of confinements in hospitals or related institutions; treatments recommended by physicians but conducted by physiotherapists, social workers, and psychologists, and so forth.

The claim should be also substantiated with receipts from pharmacists who have sold the prescribed medicines to the claimant. Receipts from nurses and attendants should also be submitted. The doctor should state the necessity for the claimants to use taxi cabs or arrive at the doctor's office with assistance.

In addition, the doctor should give a detailed history based on the report given to him by the patient, which should not contradict statements by the patient in his original application, unless the discrepancy is explained in the current report. (For instance, the patient may have recovered a previously lost memory since the first application or may not have stated an event because no one asked him.) The doctor must provide a medical report, explaining the current condition of the patient as compared with the previous finding, paying special attention to the exacerbating of the ailment as a late sequel of the persecution. The report must also include a prognosis based on findings. If a medical condition exists that is not within the scope of the reporting physician's specialty, an independent report of another physician has to be attached. If the stress due to persecution contributes to a physical illness, this has to be described and explained by the psychiatrist. If current events triggered the exacerbation, it must be shown that the patient was particularly vulnerable to such experiences due to their connection to the persecution (children leaving home, a policeman giving a ticket, a fire in the patient's house or nearby, etc.).

3. Editor's note [CK]: This was true in 1991 and pertained to the restitution and indemnification program of the former West Germany, the Federal Republic of Germany. Under communist rule, East Germany, the German Democratic Republic, had no program of indemnification. Since the unification of Germany, the German government has made it possible for former German-Jewish citizens who resided in the East German regions before their deportation or emigration to file claims for their lost property. This has turned out to be an extremely complex process, not so much as in the past by ill will, as by the fact that the Jewish properties were taken over first by German non-Jews, then confiscated by the communist regime, which rented to citizens who lived in and made improvements in the houses for over forty years. The process is incomplete as of this writing (1996). Indemnification for health-related loss of income is a moot point for all practical purposes: At this time, almost none of the adult Holocaust survivors in East Germany remain alive.

4. Paul Matussek, *Internment in Concentration Camps and its Consequences* (New York: Springer Verlag, 1975); W. Baeyer, H. Hafner, and K. P. Kisker, *Psychiatrie der Verfolgten* (Psychiatry of the persecuted) (Berlin; Springer Verlag, 1964); R. Lempp, *Extrembelastung im Kinder und Jugendalter* (Extreme burdens in childhood and youth) (Bern-Stuttgart: Hans Huber, 1979).

5. Milton Kestenberg, "Discriminatory Aspects of the German Indemnification Policy: A Continuation of Persecution," in *Generations of the Holocaust*, ed. Martin S. Bergmann and Milton E. Jucovy (New York: Basic Books, 1982), 62–79.

6. Milton Kestenberg, "The Effects of Interviews on Child Survivors," Presentation at the International Psychohistorical Association (The Graduate Center of the City University of New York), June 8, 1990.

7. Editor's note [CK]: In this case, the interviewer asked a leading question based on his knowledge and a hunch. Fortunately, he did not contaminate the data by insisting; the respondent immediately confirmed his hunch with such spontaneity that there can be no doubt that this was a genuine (not false) recovered memory. (See Kestenberg, "The Effects of Interviews on Child Survivors"; and Charlotte Kahn, "The Crossroad Between Research and Therapy," in *Children During the Nazi Reign: Psychological Perspective on the Interview Process*, ed. Judith S. Kestenberg and Eva Fogelman (Westport, Conn.: Praeger, 1994).

8. Suggested to me by Dr. Charles Fisher.

9. At the time of this writing (1991), we have not heard the answer to our petition, which was endorsed by the University of Hanover and voted upon in a plenary session.

6

Impact on the Second and Third Generations

Eva Fogelman

INTRODUCTION

In recent years, Americans have shown renewed interest in ethnic identity, personal roots, gender identity, and in symptoms-related identities such as sexually abused children and adult children of alcoholics. This has influenced a parallel development in the popularity of such specifically identified groups meeting to share their feelings and common concerns.

The identifiable groups in society, including children of alcoholics, Vietnam veterans, sexually abused women, children of survivors, and others, have been subjected to having a host of symptoms and labels attributed to all members of the group. Exposure to negative stereotyping by misinformed professionals and lay people further stigmatizes individual members in these groups who, paradoxically, join a group with a particular focus in order to feel support and a decrease in isolation and alienation.

Colleagues and friends who know of my work with generations of the Holocaust, often say, "Oh, that must be very depressing," or, "Don't you think all children of survivors are crazy?" The other day a journalist told me she wrote an article about the abnormal rate of vaginitis among children of survivors, and a noted sex therapist opined that children of survivors have more sexual problems than others. Such comments are indicative of false premises that all children of survivors are clinically depressed, anxious, and paranoid. Mental health professionals are not immune from clichés and often remark, "I have a child of survivors in treatment and is he messed up! They all are."

It is a given that patients who seek out a sex therapist have sexual problems. To then infer that all children of survivors have more sexual problems than their peers from a non-Holocaust background is an illogical next step, absent a major, controlled population study. Such a study has not been conducted. In that regard, it might be interesting to analyze those children of survivors who have sexual problems and to explore whether there is any conscious and unconscious connection to the parents' Holocaust trauma. For example, "Are female children of survivors frigid if they fantasize that their mothers survived because of sexual favors?"

Similarly, it does not follow that children of survivors who seek psychological or psychiatric treatment because they are in pain, suffering from one symptom or another, are more psychologically impaired than are their peers who are in treatment. Control studies by the late Hillel Klein and Uri Last on large controlled samples in Israel indicate that children of survivors exhibit the same degree of emotional adjustment as do their controls.[1] However, when children of survivors do suffer severe pathology, such as psychoses or schizophrenia, clinicians have observed that the onset of problems is connected to anniversary reactions or to the age of parents' traumatization, and that symptoms are Holocaust related, for example, starving, hiding in the closet (the way a parent hid during the war), putting themselves in dangerous situations, and other symptoms designed to test their capacity to survive.[2]

When Leon and her team of researchers in Minnesota employed the MMPI (Minnesota Multiple Personality Inventory), they found no differences in personality factors between children of survivors and a control group of American Jews the same age.[3] These results were confirmed by Sigal and Weinfeld, who asked hundreds of questions in a controlled study in Montreal that revealed no such differences.[4]

PSYCHOLOGICAL IMPACT OF MASSIVE TRAUMA ON SECOND AND THIRD GENERATIONS

The psychological impact of massive psychic trauma on the second and third generations—the children of survivors and their children—cannot be measured by personality tests. Rather, there is a psychological process that all children of survivors consciously or unconsciously experience, similar to the Oedipal complex in the development of sexual identity—"second generation survivor complex."[5]

Children of survivors do not experience a personality syndrome such as a posttraumatic stress disorder. By that I mean that they are not more depressed, anxious, or paranoid than a comparative cohort group. However, their development is punctuated by experiencing a mourning process they undergo, knowingly or unknowingly. Additionally, they confront very specific dynamics in communicating with their survivor parents. The mourning process and communication patterns influence their identity, interpersonal relations, and world-view. In other words, the effects on the second generation are multidimensional, especially regarding the relationship between the two psychological processes of identity formation and mourning.

Most children of survivors are named after a relative who was killed or gassed or died of disease and starvation during the Nazi persecution. Such facts are often the driving force in the identity formation of a child of survivors. While most Jews name their children after a dead member of the family, for many children of survivors their name symbolizes "victimhood." Often, living survivors interact with second generation individuals as if they, in fact, were that dead relative whose name they are carrying. A child of survivors may feel heavily burdened when carrying the name of his or her ancestor in an implicit, unspoken injunction to live that person's life in addition to his or her own. Although most times living a double life is unconscious, it can manifest itself consciously.

Children of survivors may or may not have been given information about the person whose name they are bearing. They may be living out fantasies of whom they are supposed to represent to their mother, father, or other close relative. This double-life phenomenon may manifest itself in two careers or in inconsistent behavior, such as maintaining strict religious observance when one no longer has faith (because one is supposed to be Uncle Moshe), but living a very irreligious life style when others are not noticing. Certain of these behaviors may be in harmony with their ideals and perceptions of themselves; others may be out of tune and feel strange.

Behavioral manifestations stemming from a child-of-survivor's namesake are also exacerbated by other family members' interaction with the person. Rosalie, a single woman in her twenties, expresses the burden of her confusing roles when she states in *Breaking the Silence*, "I am named after my mother's mother who was gassed in Auschwitz. I have been told I look like her, I talk like her, I sing like her. I am supposed to be my mother's mother."[6] Exasperated, she tries to save herself, to be herself. She asks, then answers, her own question: "What am I supposed to do. I couldn't take not being able to be myself, so I left when I was sixteen."

To facilitate self-differentiation and an identity integration, the conflicts, defenses, and unconscious mechanisms that develop in relation to one's name must be considered. An additional and crucial dimension to understanding the children-of-survivors' relationship to their names is the stage of mourning they are experiencing. A great many have mourned only incompletely "and this does not constitute pathology, but rather a lifetime response to massive losses, encompassing a whole world" of people and things, and an uncertainty of one's own position in that world. "Perhaps mourning of one generation is not enough and it has to continue for many generations to come."[7]

MOURNING THE LOSSES

Most experts on generations of the Holocaust agree that children of survivors, and most likely their children, continue to mourn along with the survivor generation.[8] One avenue to the understanding of this process is to become aware of how children of survivors live out their namesake's, the Holocaust victim's, life. For example, when children of survivors are asked after whom they are named and they do not know, they are presumably still in the denial stage of mourning. Such children of survivors have not begun to confront the family losses. Other forms of lack of acceptance are manifested by a change of name, either to Americanize it or to Hebraize it from the original.

When children of survivors begin the "confrontation stage" of mourning the losses and suffering of their parents, they will begin to inquire about that suffering. They may also become interested in other family members, the intergenerational family history, and the losses in the family. The work of mourning inevitably evokes feelings of guilt, sadness, depression, anger, rage, and a wish to undo the parents' suffering and helplessness.

The final stage of mourning is a beginning acceptance and, ultimately, a search for meaning. Feelings are then channeled into some meaningful action to prevent further victimization for oneself and others. Behavioral manifestations of this stage may take the form of creative expressions in art, film, writing, music, dance, or in the theater. These creations tend to reflect a remembrance of persecution or of the life that was destroyed, or a desire to teach others about what happened. Helping currently oppressed groups, bringing Nazi war criminals to trial, implementing educational and commemorative institutions, building bridges toward reduction of prejudice, and promoting tolerance are all topics of their concern.

The mourning process is impeded when a child of survivors is in a state of "transposition . . . an organizing agency which arises from the survival complex of generations. . . ." Those who experienced neither the "profound physical deterioration of ghettos and camps and the stressful conditions in hiding" may go back in time to explore their parents' pasts. "[I]n their fantasies, they live during the Holocaust and transpose the present into the past. . . . Children of survivors somatize their anxieties and depressions when they go down into the tunnel of their parents' and grandparents' existence. . . . A starving child of survivors experiences the physical feelings that go with it without knowing that she reenacts the hunger of her parents or relatives."[9]

IDENTIFICATION WITH SUFFERING

Some children of survivors are unable to mourn for their parents' suffering. Instead, they are unconsciously living as if, in the structure of their current life, they were under the Nazi occupation. Therefore, they may be suffering from an overidentification with suffering. They may be unable to enjoy themselves and experience guilt over not having suffered. They may also feel frustrated about their inability to undo the past or to get revenge, and are overwhelmed by anger and rage. Some place themselves in dangerous situations they must survive. They hide or disguise their Jewishness and become involved in oppressor-victim relationships. Thus, feeling like a victim takes on greater meaning for children of survivors.

This overidentification with the suffering has consequences in many aspects of their lives. They have difficulty trusting in relationships and are wary of making a commitment to a relationship. Possibly they choose a mate who needs to be rescued so they can feel helpful and escape the ineffectual feelings experienced in trying to undo their parents' painful past.

The connection of symptoms, defenses, wishes, and coping strategies associated with living a double life, during the Holocaust and in the present, may seem obvious to an experienced professional, but this relationship is not necessarily conscious to the child of survivors. Therefore, Holocaust-related explanations, where appropriate, could lift what is masked as depression.

Children of survivors can become aware that they are not allowing themselves to enjoy life because they think it would be disloyal to their dead relatives who suffered so much. It is important for them to realize that the dead are not expecting their descendants to "sit shiva" for them (maintain an active stance of mourning) for the rest of their lives. Such insights can provide permission to live in the present without the constant burden of living in the past as well.

DIFFERENTIATION, INTEGRATION, AND THE SEARCH FOR MEANING

The trigger for mourning the parents' suffering may be a current loss or a situation in which the person felt like a victim just once too often. This current need to cope with survival is then associated with the death of Holocaust victims in the family.

The mourning process is not a static state. It does not preclude the possibility that suddenly a new loss may bring on an old feeling, even after mourning seemingly has been completed.

In the final stage of mourning—the search for meaning—children of survivors feel a sense of integration within themselves and differentiation from others, including family members. Hence, they are less overwhelmed with their Holocaust family background. Their identity now encompasses all aspects of themselves—gender, sexual, professional, religious, and social identities—and is no longer confined to the "Holocaust self." Intense feelings are channeled into action, such as discharging moral responsibilities and creative endeavors. Such activities take place in the realm of Holocaust education, research projects, films, books, visual and performing art projects, assistance to other oppressed groups, and in the escalation of political activity, including action against Nazi war criminals and anti-Reagan demonstrations protesting his Bitburg trip. Many educational and commemorative projects were, in fact, started by children of Holocaust survivors.

The relationship between identity formation and the process of mourning experienced by children of Holocaust survivors may have a parallel in members of other second generations of victimized populations. The difference between the children of other victimized populations and the children of Holocaust survivors is that the Holocaust victims were persecuted for the mere reason that they were Jews. Hence, the process of identity formation is particularly stressful for children of Jewish Holocaust survivors. It is, therefore, of utmost importance for Jewish children of survivors to explore their feelings about their identity as Jews and resolve the attendant conflicts and confusions, particularly the idea that being Jewish is synonymous with being a victim.

THE GROUP EXPERIENCE

Through membership in a support group, or a psychotherapy group, children of survivors may find their own way to identify with the life and values that were destroyed, instead of maintaining a loyalty to the suffering. Groups reduce the isolation and normalize the feelings and attitudes that, when faced alone, seem abnormal.

As a group, children of survivors are heterogeneous. Although most are high professional achievers, having earned at least a college education, they are not overwhelmingly in the helping profession, as they are so often stereotyped. Religiously, their diversity ranges from Hassidism to Buddhism.

When young adults are members of a group whose admission criterion is having at least one parent who experienced persecution under the Nazi rule from 1933 to 1945, they provide one another with support to confront their past, encouragement to communicate with their parents and other loved ones in new ways, and alternatives to express their religious, ethnic, or national identity.

For many children of survivors, the group serves as the extended family of which they were deprived by the Nazis.

THE THIRD GENERATION

To date, systematic research on the third generation is sparse. Rosenthal and Rosenthal reported on a case study of a seven-year old whose grandmother was a Holocaust survivor.[10] They concluded that the patient suffered from existential crisis-stress syndrome and identity formation problems resulting from an identification with the grandmother. On a broader scale, fifty-one second generation families were investigated to explore the effects of the Holocaust across three generations; of these, twenty-four families had only one spouse who was a child of survivors. Twelve non-Holocaust families served as controls.[11] In this study, parents and teachers were asked questions only about the oldest child of the third-generation family. The results revealed a familial-survivor syndrome consisting of depression, anxiety, aggression, social withdrawal, feelings of loss, fearfulness, guilt, and psychosomatic complaints.

In Montreal, a survey of clinical and nonclinical third-generation people found them to be functioning better than the control group on items such as: warm, affectionate, happy, good mood, friendly, self-confident, peaceful, and easy-going.[12] Clinical evidence showed no differences between grandchildren of survivors and the control group on mood, personality, or behavior items.[13]

To understand the effects on the third generation, researchers and clinicians cannot look for answers to a personality syndrome. Bienstock, who interviewed three generations of female survivors and similar controls, concluded that the third generation communicated much better with the grandparent generation than did the second generation with their Holocaust-survivor parents.[14] The relationship between survivor grandparents and their grandchildren was warmer and closer than in the control pairs.

The third generation needs to be understood in the context of their lives. Problems in relation to the Holocaust may arise if their parents or grandparents choose to tell them the gory details of persecution and loss. Sometimes children of survivors, in the thirties-to-forties age bracket with a newly found interest in the Holocaust, want to make sure that their children learn about the Holocaust at an early age. The parents may start talking about it to their offspring as early as age three, even before the children ask any questions. These second-generation parents, wanting to spare their children the conspiracy of silence they felt growing up, unfortunately totally ignore the age-appropriateness of their communications.

Grandchildren may reevoke in the survivors the loss of their children during the war and may unconsciously trigger a mourning state and an inappropriately overprotective role toward these grandchildren, who are growing up in a different context.

If second-generation members have not successfully worked through the inner-personal dynamics of growing up with Holocaust-survivor parents, they may transmit their unresolved problems to their own children.

CONCLUSION

Holocaust survivors who remained silent in order to spare their own children the pain and suffering they endured are often surprised to find out that their adult children have to contend with their own psychological dynamics. Knowing details of the family's losses and persecution facilitates the inevitable mourning process that the second generation of survivors experience. The development of open communication with survivor parents enables children of survivors to come to terms with a painful legacy, to integrate it into their identity and not make it their total identity. Knowing details about their dead relatives enables the children of survivors to liberate themselves from identifying with the destructive pain, suffering, and victimization. Then they have an opportunity to identify with life-affirming facets of the deceased and to remember the dead for their strengths.

NOTES

1. Uri Last and Hillel Klein, "Impact of Parental Holocaust Traumatization on Offsprings' Reports of Parental Child-rearing Practices," *Journal of Youth and Adolescence* 4 (1984): 267–83.

2. Sylvia Axelrod, Ophilia Schnipper, and John Rau, "Hospitalized Offspring of Holocaust Survivors," *Bulletin of the Menninger Clinic* 44 (1980): 1–14.

3. Gloria R. Leon, James N. Butcher, Max Kleinman, Alan Goldberg, and Moshe Almagor, "Survivors of the Holocaust and Their Children: Current Status and Adjustment," *Journal of Personality and Social Psychology* 41 (1981): 198, 503–16.

4. John Sigal and Morton Weinfeld, *Trauma and Rebirth: International Effects of the Holocaust* (New York: Praeger, 1989).

5. Judith S. Kestenberg, "Transposition Revisited: Clinical, Therapeutic, and Developmental Considerations," in *Healing Their Wounds: Psychotherapy with Holocaust Survivors and Their Families*, ed. Paul Marcus and Alan Rosenberg (New York: Praeger, 1989), 67–82.

6. Eva Fogelman and Edward Mason (Producers), *Breaking the Silence: The Generation After the Holocaust* (New York: Cinema Guild, 1984).

7. Judith S. Kestenberg, "Coping with Losses and Survival," in *Loss and Mourning: Psychoanalytic Perspectives*, ed. David R. Dietrich and Peter C. Shabad (Madison, Conn.: International Universities Press, 1989), 402.

8. Kestenberg, "Coping."

9. Kestenberg, "Transposition," 71–72.

10. P. A. Rosenthal and S. Rosenthal, "Holocaust Effects in the Third Generation: Child of Another Time," *American Journal of Psychotherapy* 34, no. 4 (1980): 572–80.

11. Israel Rubenstein, "Multigenerational Occurrences of Survivorsyndrome Symptoms in Families of Hocolcaust Survivors," Unpublished Doctoral Dissertation, California School of Professional Psychology, Fresno, 1981.

12. Sigal and Weinfeld, *Trauma and Rebirth*.

13. Ibid. One of the clinical defenses manifested was identifying with the aggressor, and two prevalent symptoms were a high degree of fear and eating problems.

14. Bonnie Bienstock, "Daughters and Granddaughters of Female Concentration Camp Survivors: Mother-Daughter Relationship" (Unpublished Doctoral Dissertation, Florida Institute of Technology, 1988).

7

Antisemitism and Jewish Identity in Hungary Between 1989 and 1994*

Judit Mészáros

INTRODUCTION

The democratic transformation of the ex-communist states of central Europe is a historically unique phenomenon that raises a number of interesting social, political, sociological, and intrapsychic questions.

It is not easy to present a realistic picture of a relatively brief, but very intensive era, especially when we ourselves remain subject to its processes. The five-year-long period is not a "past"; it actually belongs to our contemporary time. To jump over the distance between the microworld of psychic events and the macroworld of social movements surrounding the individual implies further difficulties for the psychotherapist or psychoanalyst. For these reasons, it seems appropriate to begin by assembling certain of the writings of my colleagues—historians, sociologists, and psychotherapists—who have, in the field of Jewish identity, contributed to the exploration, description, and interpretation of social and psychological processes. Based on their work and on my own experience, I have attempted to outline the most marked features and changes of the past five years, with no claim to completeness, but with the aim of providing a useful survey of the field. To interpret contemporary phenomena, however, one must first recall some important events of an earlier past.

HISTORICAL BACKGROUND

In the twentieth century, central Europe has witnessed a great number of sharp historic turns. In the seven decades since World War I, Hungary has

*Translated by Bea Ehmann.

undergone seven switches of the political regime. Comparing the history of the country to that of other European countries reveals that Hungarian political public life in the modern era has shown unusually large oscillations between the extremes of philosemitism and antisemitism.[1]

Nineteenth-century enlightenment and emancipation had brought about fundamental changes in the social role of Hungarian Jewry. Many Jews had unambiguously supported the efforts of the liberal nobility to modernize Hungary. Assimilated Hungarian Jews clearly identified themselves as Hungarian nationals even while remaining "Israelites" in terms of their religious affiliation. In previous centuries, Hungary had been the most tolerant of Jews among the countries of this region, and Jews believed they were well integrated into the society. This strong tendency to assimilate was expressed by the widespread changing of German-sounding family names into Hungarian ones, for example, Löwinger into Lukacs, Fränkel into Ferenczi. The adaptive efforts of assimilating Jewry had specific cultural parallels as well. For example, while earlier the small synagogues tended to be placed in inner yards of buildings, the assimilated upper middle class of Pest built a synagogue, the largest functioning synagogue in Europe, accommodating some 3,000 people, and, surprisingly, is equipped with a musical instrument typical of Christian churches, an organ.

By the end of the nineteenth century, Hungarian Jewry enjoyed equality under the law and in economics and religion. They played an important role in the processes of capital formation and cultural modernization. However, the liberal state of the Dualism—the Austro-Hungarian Monarchy after the Compromise of 1867—was unable to solve the burning societal problems, especially the social difficulties and the question of nationalities. New political tendencies had evolved in the form of bourgeois radical and socialist ideas. The end of World War I, followed by an immediate Bourgeois Revolution and Commune, brought a crisis not only to the liberal state, but also to the radical and social bourgeoisie, which had a great number of Jewish citizens in their ranks. Pogroms and political antisemitism appeared again in the twenties.

Unfortunately, Hungary became the first among the European societies in the twentieth century to pass discriminatory legislation such as the numerus clausus, which limited the number of Jewish students at the universities. How could it have happened that the Hungarian government codified anti-Jewish laws between 1938 and 1943? The aim of early anti-Jewish laws was to keep Jews out of the mainstream of social life; the later ones focused on forfeiture of Jewish property. Years before the German occupation, recent Jewish immigrants to Hungary who did not have the benefit of citizenship were deported to the concentration camp at Kamenec-Podolsk. When the Nazis came to power and Hungary was occupied by German troops, the overt aim was complete physical extermination. The Hungarian authorities and the majority of the population cooperated with the German occupiers and contributed to the annihilation of about half-a-million and the deportation of the majority of the Hungarian Jews.

This naturally implies that the remaining Hungarian Jewry saw the Soviet Army as their rescuers. It appeared as if the Red Army in Hungary meant their very survival. For the survivors, the new political regime necessarily represented something different from what it signified to the gentile citizens of the country: the possibility of a society without discrimination. Jews who survived the Holocaust had either not returned to the country that had brought its discriminated-against citizens to the death camps, or had left the country soon after coming back from the camps. Those who did remain in the country tried to start a new life. Following the three years of a coalition government after the war, power was seized by the Communist Party, which ruled with dictatorial methods from 1948 onward. Under the new regime, new possibilities opened for the surviving Jews who remained in Hungary, since it was a basic precondition that the reorganized power structures of the new political system would be open only to people who had not compromised themselves under the former regime. Therefore, Jews who had been persecuted earlier now wholly satisfied this precondition, and were allowed to occupy previously unimaginable positions in the governmental administration and in the army. These jobs had previously been open only to members of the gentile nobility and, since before World War I, to the middle class. However, immediately after World War I, the anti-Jewish laws of the Horthy regime had provided legal guarantees for the exclusion of Jews from these positions.

What was promised and demanded by the new regime was ambitious: the safety of a society creating complete equality—the end of the Jewish question, antisemitism, and national isolation, and an end to all kinds of class stratification, which meant a great deal to the previously outlawed and persecuted Jews who survived the *Shoah*.[2] Many of them found new meaning for life in humanistic ideas and in the Communist movement as a substitute for their destroyed families and lost relatives.

From those to whom the promises were addressed, the Communist Party required complete identification with the "movement." For the bourgeois-intellectual Jew, meeting this demand actually meant giving up the self as a whole: renouncing previous personality patterns, behavioral habits, ways of thinking, and education. All these were labeled as unacceptable "remnants of [a] bourgeois past."[3] Naturally, this also implied the rejection of Jewishness as a history and an identity.[4] On the other hand, this meant that it became possible for Jews to launch a hopeful new life in a discrimination-free world, and that they could rid themselves of the persecuted Jewish past forthwith. The price to be paid for this privilege was to forego the opportunity to work through their trauma, inasmuch as they had to deny their past or at least remain silent about it.

This was the point at which the psychological process came to a standstill and a paradox developed that for decades proved to be an inescapable source of intrapsychic and interpersonal conflicts. Thus, an anxiety-laden world of taboos, silences, and discontinuous life histories evolved.

At the societal level, not dealing with the past seemed to be advantageous insofar as it protected the Hungarian society from having to face the anti-Jewish measures enacted between 1920 and 1944. Hungarians thus could ignore the responsibility both for some citizens' active participation in the deportation of the Jews and the majority's compliant indifference. Silence also served the interests of the ruling party, which tried to avoid the tension evoked by the prejudice "Communism means Jewish rule."

Although based on actual interest patterns, this process created only a short-term state of equilibrium between the contracting parties. On a long-term basis it both induced and concealed pathological processes.

PSYCHOLOGICAL CONSEQUENCES

Global denial, neglect of the past, "redefining" life events of individuals, and the effort to repress the traumata served social adaptation. This accommodation to the new situation at the level of a societal consensus soon produced psychological symptoms. Lasting for more than forty years, this frozen state was followed by a melting process in the seventies and eighties. Some researchers and psychotherapists became curious about what happened to the survivors and to the children of survivors during this period. What happens in a society where the past had been categorized as a taboo? Would the absence of "fathers" have hindered an optimal development for the next generation even without the taboo?

There were few people in the surviving families who could pass on traditions. This situation was exacerbated by the anticlerical attitude of the political regime, which limited the institutional function of the churches and restricted practice of the Jewish religion. Anyone suitable to pass on tradition had to face the fact that he or she was unable to offer a positive model for identification since being a Jew entailed the stigmatized, anxiety-provoking experience of being a member of an endangered group. Embracing a Jewish identity became almost equivalent to identifying with martyrdom. In any case, identifying positively with a group that radiates joylessness is hardly possible, even in the absence of other hindrances. A further barrier to identity development in post–World War II Hungarian children was the great number of mixed marriages. The unworked-through traumas of the surviving parents, the decades-long silences, the attempts to rewrite the past, and the restrictions on religion and tradition all brought about major psychological consequences in the succeeding generations.

The most characteristic manifestations of the psychological sequelae discerned during the past decade are the discovery of identity confusions, the unconscious transfer of parental trauma to the next generation, the second-and third-generation (survivor) syndrome, and dramatic disclosures of "how I came to realize that I was Jewish."[5]

CHANGE OF POLITICAL REGIME AND FACING THE REMINISCENCES OF THE PAST

Several metaphors have been offered to illustrate the dynamics of the change of the political regime. Some authors claimed it was like a refrigerator that had frozen our history, and as a function of the melting process, the national, ethnic, and political ideas of the twenties and thirties are gradually exposed to view as they emerge from the ice blocks.[6] Another possible metaphor is that of the genie in the bottle, who creates a storm while freeing himself. Other images illustrate dramatic manifestations such as irrationality or the anxiety-provoking force of repressed negative emotions and prejudices, which, bound to the past, are evoked by present-day events.

The above metaphors capture what cannot be avoided at either the individual or the societal level. The sources of irrational outcomes can be found in the denied past, the consciously garbled or repressed past, the unelaborated individual, and in ethnic and social tensions—all intertwined with present events.

In the years preceding the change of political regime in Hungary, "overt antisemitism was still perceived as a sign of political bad taste."[7] After the latest change of regime, political antisemitism appeared again, in the 1990 election campaign. It was directed mostly against the liberal Free Democrats, and in the form of anonymous street posters and throw-away leaflets. Soon afterward, a writer-politician declaring openly anti-Semitic views emerged. Istvan Csurka[8], cloaked in the colors of the governing party, the Hungarian Democratic Forum, announced that "Free Democrats are a violent minority" seeking to seize power in the country by methods learned from Karl Marx and Gyorgy Lukacs.[9] Hungarians of national-popular roots have to be protected from the influence of a "pigmy minority."[10] The Antall government did not reject this opinion and implicitly approved the nationalistic rhetoric reminiscent of the years preceding World War II. With this, anti-Semitic manifestations found a national forum. Anti-Jewish utterances became an everyday phenomenon in Hungary. It is interesting to observe the further stages of this process and to recognize the stereotypes of the 1920s and 1930s in the contents of these prejudices. Another leader of the governmental party, this time a poet, Sandor Csoori, wrote in a right-wing journal, "Liberal Hungarian Jewry intends to 'assimilate' the Hungarians to their style and thinking. For this, they have made themselves a parliamentary platform larger than ever before."[11] In reply, several members of the governmental and public personages raised a protest, and Arpad Goncz, president of the Republic, denounced the poet-politician. Nevertheless, the newly regenerated anti-Semitic wave has continued to grow and has attacked even Arpad Goncz, who was decried by Csurka as "an agent of Communists and reform-Communists, Paris, New York, and Tel Aviv liaisons."[12] In these excerpts, it is not difficult to recognize the enduring phraseology of fear and hatred of the presumed "world-power aspirations of the cosmopolitan-bolshevik, rootless Jewry." As a response, the democratic-minded segment of the society expressed their indignation in the form of a silent street demonstration. At the time of the reemergence of publicly articulated prejudices, a woman who survived the Holocaust at the age of nine was interviewed. Her parents also survived the Holocaust and preserved their bourgeois-Jewish values. The child, never refuting her Jewish identity, started to work enthusiastically for the building of the new society. At the beginning, she believed in the possibility of a discrimination-free social system. During the interview she said, "When about 30 years ago, I thought that we have to go ahead and make a career at any rate. [But] my father would always say: 'It is not good to be so agitated in the foreground; you should not do so. Go and stay in the background, on the third line. It is not good; they do not like it. There is Gero, there is Rakosi, Revai, this is no good to anybody.'[13] At that time, I was far from agreeing with him. But today I see that, as in many other things, he was absolutely right. There is no need to be a busybody up front. I myself am ambivalent about the Free Democrats[14] and their allies being in the limelight in front of everyone. There are moments when I think they had better give back this country to those who are at home here." In these words, it is not difficult to recognize the tendency of identification with the anti-Semitic discriminative prejudices, and to see its paralyzing power.

Concurrently with these events, psychotherapists began to ask one another, "Are everyday politics appearing in your sessions as well?" We were facing a new phenomenon. Social tension had entered the consulting room. I was suspicious even earlier, noticing that during the repressive years of the past, it was not usual to speak about political, ideological, or religious issues in the psychotherapeutic situation, not even on the psychoanalytic couch. As an analyst colleague of mine admitted, "I was really deaf to this problem." We may suppose that an entire generation has grown up avoiding the elaboration of political and family-root conflicts in their analyses or any other therapy, and facing them truly only when the whole society started to "melt." One of the best-known researchers in Hungary, who started to conduct interviews very early, at the beginning of the eighties, speaks as follows: "Now I do not have any severe identity problems. I must say it has developed parallel with my interview work, with thinking about it, with the related dialogues. I would constantly compare the interviewees' answers to my own possible ones, and this, in turn, helped me to clarify many of my viewpoints as to previously unanswered questions. The starting point was only blindness, not any kind of certainty."[15]

Prejudice in Hungary in the 1990s

We now know a lot about the causes of this "deafness" and "blindness," and also about why it was no longer possible to ignore political currents and prejudiced thinking in the course of psychotherapies in the nineties. I would think frequently about how therapists—Jewish or not—might respond to explicit, crude anti-Semitic utterances. I wondered how they handle their countertransference feelings; how they react to the outburst of their harshly anti-Semitic patients; how they try to translate social prejudices into the language of intrapsychic dynamics. Where are the limits of neutrality? Should the therapist (who is annoyed by a patient's antisemitism) tell her patient (who harbors the deliberate intention to irritate the therapist) that she is a Jew, thereby allowing the exploration of sadomasochistic dynamics? And, in this context, should jealousy be explored, involving new stereotypes such as, "I want to be like the Jews, clever, different, powerful." On the other hand, the patient deeply despises the Jews, the "excluders," who help only each other and take part in a worldwide conspiracy.

In one particular patient's fantasy, everybody who is better and more talented than he is a Jew. He purposely chose a Jewish analyst, went to work in a bank (thereby choosing a "Jewish profession"), and bought an apartment in a district once labeled as "Jewish" (and is convinced that the house is populated only with Jews, even at present). The patient has been in negative transference with his Jewish analyst for years, and one wonders how to evaluate his fantasy that, in case of a new persecution of the Jews, he would give shelter to her. Certainly, one thing should not, and cannot be done: to remain "deaf."

However, hearing, perceiving, becoming aware of denied, garbled, or simply repressed events, when the force of external reality breaks through the wall of ego defense mechanisms, will unavoidably lead to feelings of pain, fear, and anxiety. And exactly this has happened when making use of false notions of freedom such as, "today we are free to do everything" and "political antisemitism gained its civil rights" in the budding democracy of Hungary.

An outstanding professor of history fulminated at an international conference held to commemorate the fiftieth anniversary of the Holocaust:

> During the past years, leading public personalities . . . have made anti-Jewish utterances fit for good society. The government . . . while trying to make excuses against the not at all unfounded accusation of antisemitism, has regularly failed to take measures—at least by enforcing the prevailing laws—against overt or covert anti-Semitic incitements, and for a short time, it even took the instigators under protection . . . and what it has not done at all was to take a role in historical clarification, in honest elucidation of the situation . . . there are some who even make strong efforts to employ the Arrow-Cross [Hungarian

Nazi Party] phraseology . . . or create new codes: "cosmopolitan, liberal, Western value system," etc., all these have become smear-words, euphemisms for a world "Jew."[16]

Broad social strata were frustrated by the misinterpretation of democracy, by the victory of libertarianism over liberty. Citizens who are members of minority groups, who are seen as "other"—the Jew, the Gypsy, the Arab— no longer feel safe. Many speak of their anxieties. For example, a woman who was severely abused in a *Gestapo* prison said, "in recent weeks, I have been suffering from insomnia. When I go to sleep, I have nightmares and wake up all in a sweat." To the questions why her anxieties have been renewed, she replied with just a name: "Csurka."[17] What does this name represent, and how has it gained a symbolic meaning? The answer is very simple. At that time, the bearer of this name belonged to the social elite and to the government. History shows that antisemitic forces can achieve significant influence only if they gain the approval of the social elite, or at a minimum, if they do not meet resistance from that quarter. During the rule of a government that, after having been elected democratically, shifted to the right, this fear was likely to be realized. It is not difficult, therefore, to understand why the patient invoked the name of a writer-politician with a leading role in the governing party as an explanation for her anxious state.

Whenever the social elite consciously rejects antisemitic ideas, it is highly unlikely that antisemitism will entail serious danger. But if the elite fails to do so (as the government of John Antall failed to take measures in due time) then the vulnerable citizen may well lose his feelings of comfort and safety. Here we have to state explicitly that the first Hungarian government freely elected after the collapse of the Soviet Bloc in 1989 made a severe error in not taking timely measures with sufficient force against the reappearance of antisemitic manifestations. As a result, racist prejudices and xenophobia intensified, and skinhead groups emerged. Certain members of Parliament protected the groups that, under the banner of nationalism, verbally attacked Arabs, Jews, and Gypsies, wildly shouting extreme right-wing epithets. Subsequently, protest groups, committed to democratic ideas, emerged. This can be viewed as a sign of the self-protective power of society.

A Survey of Prevailing Attitudes

A question may rightfully be posed regarding the degree to which racism and antisemitism are present in Hungary in the 1990s. Though no sociological studies covering the whole population have been conducted in recent years, sociologists have conducted some surveys among university students. And since the behavior of the social elite is a very important determinant of prejudiced thinking in society, the results of this study may be considered to have significance.

In the course of this study, a survey was made of 1,000 college and university students in Hungary.[18] This sample represents the complete range of Hungarian students with respect to age, sex, geographic locations, and type of institution. The researchers mapped both the cognitive (stereotypes) and the affective and conative (situations motivating for action) dimensions of prejudiced thinking. The statements put to the responders were selected to reveal all three dimensions of prejudiced attitudes: the cognitive, affective, and conative.

The majority of the students lacked both accurate information about the number of Jews living in Hungary today and of the number killed in the Holocaust. The number of Jews living in Hungary was estimated at more than 100,000 by 80 percent of the respondents, while 20 percent estimated more than half a million. In fact, there are about 80,000 Hungarian Jews.

The number of Jews killed in the Holocaust was underestimated by 58 percent of the interviewees. More than one-third of these students (36 percent) simultaneously underestimated the number of Holocaust victims and overestimated the present size of the Jewish population in Hungary. Yet, very few think that Jews are "dirty" (4 percent), or that they "disaffect or weaken the nations which take them in."[19]

Among present-day university students, 45.7 percent are free from all kinds of antisemitic prejudice, 44.7 percent are "moderately" antisemitic, with more or less anti-Jewish prejudice; and 9.6 percent of them are hardcore antisemites.[20] The analyses indicate that while negative stereotypes and certain themes of political antisemitism are virulent among the Hungarian population, relatively few people would agree with any item that refers to some kind of discrimination or segregation.

Further orientation is possible if the degree of antisemitism in Hungary is compared to that in neighboring, ex-socialist countries. In a 1991 study by the American Jewish Committee on the attitudes toward Jews in Poland, Hungary, and Czechoslovakia, 1,200 people from each country were asked about their attitudes toward various minorities and outgroups, including Jews. The results revealed that of the three countries, more negative feelings toward Jews prevail in Poland than in either Czechoslovakia or Hungary. Czechoslovakia ranks second in this regard, with Hungary manifesting the least anti-Jewish sentiment. Within each of these countries there is far less negative feeling toward Jews than toward other groups in the society— Gypsies, former communist officials, Arabs, Russians, blacks, and so on.

Nevertheless, if we look at the figures, we find that even in relatively nonantisemitic countries, the number of respondents who do agree with various antisemitic statements is not negligible. This number rarely falls below 10 percent, and in some instances, it is strikingly high. For example, 17 percent of Hungarians would prefer not to have Jews in their neighborhood (Poland, 40 percent; Czechoslovakia, 23 percent). Somewhat fewer (12 percent) Hungarians agree with the statement that "Jews have too much influence over our country's economy" (Poland, 10 percent; Czechoslovakia, 6 percent).[21]

POSITIVE CHANGES

The results of this poll suggest that a fairly large number of Hungarians feel distanced from the Jews and share certain stereotypes regarding their influence. However, despite these negative developments, the past five years have witnessed markedly positive changes, not the least being the public apology tendered by the Hungarian Episcopates for sins against Hungarian Jewry during World War II.

Changes have also occurred within the Jewish communities, along with a greater awareness and acceptance of a Jewish identity. The great many books, journals, conferences on the Holocaust, and the often huge mass of people meeting in the restored main synagogues and community houses also indicate the arrival of a new era. Two basic processes have begun: the working through of the past and the possibility of an organized education of future generations. Consequently, children of the survivors and their children have been able to meet with each other, to take steps toward the necessary "working through," and to establish new Jewish schools that offer the possibility of connecting the latest generations to traditional Jewish education.

The process of working through started at several levels as soon as the consensual social silence melted. This process was aided by intensive interviews with the survivors and their children, and was carried out by several independent research groups including sociologists, social psychologists, and psychoanalysts.[22] The trend was supported by psychotherapeutic healing work and by groups in which survivors, their children, and grandchildren could meet and speak about the traumata of the nondisclosed or repressed past.[23] Though the number of active participants has been relatively small (only 500 altogether), these activities have resulted in a real ideological breakthrough. They have had an impact on family members and on the individuals' broader system of relationships.

In 1989–1990, for the first time in decades, two twelve-grade Jewish schools were founded in Budapest: the American Foundation School, which places greater emphasis on religious education and maintains close contact with the official religious community; and the less-religious Lauder Javne Community School. The pupils enrolled in these schools are the children of the first generation born after the Holocaust. Thus, when including the surviving grandparents, this development concerns three generations. The identity-forming function of these schools is obvious. The individual motives for this choice manifest new forms and depths of Jewish identity in Hungary.[24]

CONCLUSION

We cannot suppose that prejudiced thinking, attempts to exclude minorities, or the series of civil wars being fought on nationalist bases in our region will end soon. But we may hope that, through the means offered by democracy, through knowledge offered by the humanities and psychology, and by keeping firmly in mind the experiences of the past, the conditions necessary for free and safe development may be achieved and the destructive processes threatening such development can be controlled.

NOTES

1. Mária M. Kovács, "Zsidóság és magyarok a rendszerváltás utan" (Jews and Hungarians after the change of the political regime), in *Zsidóság-identitás-történelem (Jewishness-identity-history)*, ed. Mária M. Kovacs, Yitzhak Kashti, and Ferenc Eros, (Budapest: T-Twins, 1993), 49.

2. Hebrew word for Holocaust.

3. Péter Várdy, *"A magyarországi zsidoüldözesek a hazai tortenetírásban. Szemleti problémák és a kérdés aktualitasa"* (Persecution of the Jew in Hungary as reflected in Hungarian historical literature), in *Zsidoság az 1945 utani, Magyarországon (Jewry in Hungary after 1945)* (Paris: Magyar Füzetek, 1984), 184.

4. Peter Kende, "Bevezetō" (Introduction) in *Zsidosag az 1945 utáni Magyarországon (Jewry in Hungary after 1945)* (Paris: Magyar Füzetek, 1984), v–xv.

5. Ferenc Erōs, András Kovács, and Katalin Lévay, *"Hogyan jottem ra, hogy zsidó vagyok"* (How I came to realize I was Jewish) *Medvetanc* 2–3 (1985): 129–44; Terez Virag, "Children of the Holocaust and Their Children's Children: Working Through Trauma in the Psychotherapeutic Process," *Dynamic Psychotherapy* 2 (Spring/Summer 1984): 1; Judit Mészáros, "L'apparitions des refoulements sociaux dans une cure psychanalytique" (The specter of social oppression during a psychoanalytic treatment) in *Entre Savoir et Ignorance: le questionnement psychanalytique (Between knowledge and ignorance: The psychoanalytic query)* (Bruxelles: 1992), 4–5.

6. Lászlo Karsai, "A Shoah a magyar sajtóban 1989–91" (Shoah in the Hungarian newspapers), in *Zsidóság-identitás-történelem (Jewishness-identity-history)*, ed., Mária M. Kovács, Yitzhak Kashti, and Ferenc Erōs (Budapest: T-Twins, 1993), 59–81.

7. Mária M. Kovács, "Zsidóság és magyarok," 49.

8. István Csurka, a celebrated playwright and novelist in the communist era, became the leading figure of the Hungarian extreme right. He was originally elected to Parliament in 1990. After a long hesitation, Prime Minister Jozsef Antall decided to dismiss him in 1993. After their split, Csurka founded his own extreme-right party.

9. Hungarian Democratic Forum: founded in 1988, a right-central movement, then a party, that, achieving the best results in the first free elections in 1990, became the leading force of the governmental coalition in 1990–1994. The president of the

party was Jozsef Antall, who was the prime minister until his death in 1993. The party lost the 1994 elections and went into opposition.

10. Karsai, *"A Shoa."*

11. Sandor Csoori, "Napali Hold" (Daylight moon), *Hitel* 9 (September 1990): 5–6.

12. I. Csurka, "Néhány gondolat" (Some thoughts), *Magyar Forum* 34 (August 1992): 3.

13. Ernō Gerō, Mátyás Rákosi, and József Révai: leading Communist politicians of Jewish origin who returned to Hungary from Soviet emigration in 1944–45; responsible for unlawful actions after 1949.

14. Free Democrats: since 1988, a political party evolving from the liberal opposition movement consisting mostly of intellectuals. After the 1990 elections, the decisive force of the parliamentary opposition. The party entered into a governing coalition with the Socialist Party after the elections of 1994.

15. Szántô T. Gábor, "A zsidó szellem az európai gondolkodás kiirthatatlan része. Interjú Erōs Ferenccel" (The Jewish spirit in European thought is ineradicable. Interview with Ferenc Erōs), *Szombat* 6, no. 9 (1994):9.

16. Géza Komoróczy, "A pernye beleég bōrünkbe" (Flying ash burns into our skins), *Beszélō* (April 1994): 30.

17. Teréz Virág, "Veszkorszak és pszichológia" (Shoa and psychology), *Magyar Hirlap* (1994).

18. András Kovács, "Zsidók és magyarok. Csoportszereotipiák mai magyar egyetemisták korében" (Jews and Hungarians. Group stereotypes among the Hungarian university student today), *Világosság* 34, no. 8–9 (1993): 68–75.

19. János Gadó, "Antiszemitizmus az egyetemisták kōzōtt" (Antisemitism among university students), *Szombat* 9 (1994): 12–14.

20. Kovács, "Zsidók es magyarok."

21. Ferenc Erōs and Zoltán Fabián, *Anti-Semitism in Hungary, 1990–1994.* Manuscript. Attitudes toward Jews in Poland, Hungary, and Czechoslovakia. A comparative study for the American Jewish Committee and Freedom House, January 1991, by Penn and Schoen Associates, in cooperation with Demoskp Research Agency (Poland), Median, Inc. (Hungary), Association for Independent Social Analysis (Czechoslovakia.) See also: "Folgenkonflikte der Umwältungen in Ostmitteleuropa," *Journal für Sozialforschung* 31, no. 4 (1991); Ferenc Erōs and Zoltán Fabián, "Antisemitism in Hungary, 1990–1994," in *Jahrbuch für Antisemitismusforschung*, Werner Bergmann ed. (Frankfurt–New York: Campus Verlag, 1995), 342–56.

22. Ferenc Erōs, "Megtorni a hallgatást" (To break the silence), *Múlti és jövö. Zsidó kulurális antológia* (Past and future Jewish cultural anthologies) 2 (1988): 19–27; Judit Mészáros and Erzsébe Juhász (Interviews with child-survivors). Manuscript (in cooperation with Judith Kestenberg, Child Development Research, Sands Point, New York). István Cserne, Katalin Petō, Jŭlia Szilágyi, and György Szōke, "Az elsō és a második generáció" (The first and second generation), *Psychiatria Hungarica* 7 (1992): 2.

23. Teréz Virág, "A holocaust színdróma megjolonése a pszichoteŕapiás gyakorlatban" (Appearance of the Holocaust syndrome in psychotherapeutic practice). Manuscript, 1994.

24. Éva Kovács and Júlia Vajda, "Identitásk eresés-Iskkolaválaszás" *(Seeking identity-choosing school)*. Manuscript, 1992.

Part II

CHILDREN'S RESPONSES TO PERSECUTION

Charlotte Kahn

Children are not prepared to cope with frights beyond imagination—to be ripped from the safety of their homes, to be given away by their own parents, to live in hiding at the mercy of strangers, to have to pretend they are someone other than who they thought they were, to be hungry constantly, to witness cruelty and death. Children not only lack the benefit of "inoculation"[1] against stress and the preparedness that may reduce some adults' vulnerability to trauma; they have not even completely developed the personality structures that enable adults to cope with normal circumstances. Then how much greater is the children's traumatization under catastrophic conditions such as persecution? And how, under such conditions, are they to create their identity?

Young children who are given away lose trust in their mothers, and infants lose the benefit of the life-supporting regulation for which they rely upon their parents. This protection and regulation extends beyond physical safety to the rescuing of infants from their unfathomable terror emanating from overwhelming "somatic, preverbal, timeless, archaic affects."[2] Additionally, older children's exposure to cruelty in general, and to the victimization of their parents in particular, interferes with the idealization of their parents. Children may overidealize dead parents; but the parents' helplessness may result in devalued other- and self-images as was the case for Jehuda, who unconsciously thought of himself as a "vermin."[3] Still other reactions to victimization are "identification with the aggressor"[4] and becoming prematurely adult-like. This can be observed also in preschoolers who take care of infant siblings when their mothers are ill, absent, or deceased. Overall, the great danger for traumatized children is that the developmental process becomes fundamentally disturbed or arrested, leaving "an often hidden somatic and psychomotor component to all affects."[5]

The earlier the trauma occurs in a person's life, the more devastating the effect. Survivors who had not yet reached adulthood at the time of the onset of World War II later manifest a higher rate of psychological symptoms,[6] and very young traumatized children are at risk of suffering serious personality deviations and distortions.[7] In contrast to infants and young children, traumatized adults with an established personality may regress partially in order to survive. Though they may operate on lower levels of development with diminished or even some lost functioning, and though their ordeals often resulted in long-lasting, sometimes late-appearing, physical and psychological symptoms, their basic personality nevertheless remained intact.

Contrary to the popular belief that children have no memory of their early experiences, infant traumatic experiences are stored, albeit in sensory-motor (not semantic and conceptual) form. Unavailable to conscious recall, these early stored experiences nonetheless influence behavior, even in adulthood. By contrast, frequent, sudden terror experienced at a later age (that is, after two-and-a-half to three years old) can be rearoused by related stimuli (visual, auditory, or olfactory) and then retrieved. This is feasible because very early "affectively charged experiences" are characterized by "indelibility."[8] Unlike sudden, infrequent terror, repeated trauma is more often dealt with by denial, splitting, and dissociation, thereby becoming less accessible to consciousness, but producing symptoms such as emotional dulling, "self-anaesthesia," and nightmares. Clearly, trauma sustained even in very early childhood leaves a permanent scar on the psyche, as does adult-sustained trauma.

Regardless whether memories are nonverbal or conceptualized and split-off, they are not fully conscious, and in that state they defy mourning and integration. Consequently, such memories frequently impel survivors throughout their lives to recreate the victim and oppressor roles of the original trauma and even to act them out with their own children.[9] Thus, the effects of the Holocaust and other social and physical traumata can be transmitted multigenerationally and, thereby, perpetuated.

It is encouraging, however, that many child survivors of persecution manage to heal themselves by sharing their woes and pleasures in groups with other survivors, as well as through creative works. In the ensuing chapters, survivors, interviewers of survivors, and researchers have recorded and evaluated some persecuted children's oppression and healing.

In *Child Survivors: A Review*, Paul Valent introduces the theme of children's responses to persecution by showing that child survivors can establish a more integrated sense of self by including survivorship as part of their identity. It would seem that the process of integrating survivorship into identity can be likened to first lifting repressions and then integrating those formerly unavailable experiences and feelings into consciousness. This is, in fact, what Anna Maria Jokl's Jewish and Nazi patients did when they confronted their unconscious images of themselves as "vermin" and "beast."[10]

Valent writes that recognizing themselves as survivors makes membership in a group of child survivors possible, giving them the opportunity to reduce feelings of aloneness and inferiority. The group responses may cast a different perspective on conscious memories, enabling some survivors to replace shame with pride. Their acceptance of the lost family may foster both a sense of the historical process and the survivor's place within it. These are important aspects of living in the present, looking to the future, and appreciating the triumph over death.

Judith S. Kestenberg postulates in *Nazi Fathers* that cruel behavior (encouraged by Nazi philosophy and goals) affected many Nazis' patterns of fathering. She hypothesizes that hostile feelings toward their own children (encouraged by Germanic traditions) were at times projected outward, making atrocities against children of Jews and Gypsies emotionally acceptable. Case studies document a harsh treatment of their own offspring by some Nazi fathers. This caused several of these children to identify with the Jewish victims of the Holocaust. Kestenberg focuses on the psychological mechanisms of splitting and projection, the attitudes toward weakness and sickness, and the wall of silence around Nazi fathers' sadistic activities. She demonstrates how the idealization of strength, sacrifice, and death wishes motivated Nazi fathers.

In the following chapter, Judith S. Kestenberg discusses *The Persecution of Polish Children*, delineating distinctions between the suffering of non-Jewish and of Jewish-Polish children as a result of Nazism. Brief vignettes illustrate hardships, dilemmas, and confusions faced by children in both groups.

Yugoslavian Child-Survivors are introduced by Nikola Volf. The chapter is based on interviews with fifty Jewish Yugoslavs who, as children, lived through World War II. They reported on events of great psychological consequence, for example, the execution of their fathers, physical illnesses, lasting ailments, and their postwar dreams. They were questioned about their adaptation to the new life circumstances, including choice of spouse and attitudes of the younger generation. Volf draws attention to the social context as a strong determinant of attitudes. Jewish youths in a Yugoslavia that has lost its communist identity now look toward Judaism and Israel.

Charlotte Kahn discusses *German-Jewish Identity* from the very personal perspective of a girl who was five years old at the time the Nazis came to power, and ten years of age when she left her home following *Kristallnacht*, the Night of Broken Glass. The values and sociopsychological conditions characterizing German-Jewish identity, which strongly influenced this child survivor, are traced historically with references to the lives of prominent figures.

In the chapter *Kindertransport*, Judith S. Kestenberg informs the readers that during the time of the Nazi regime, 10,000 children were sent from Germany to England, Austria, and Czechoslovakia to escape Nazi oppression. The experiences of a seven-year-old girl reveal that, though their lives were saved, the *Kindertransport* children were spared neither the trauma of sudden separation from their parents nor the consequent shock of abandonment.

Sweden and the Holocaust, by Hedi Fried, is a bird's-eye-view historical account of Jews in Sweden since Viking times, Jewish refugees during the Nazi era, and survivors arriving immediately following World War II. For Holocaust child-survivors the psychological work of forming an integrated personality was most difficult under the conditions of physical, social, and psychological stress they had endured. Fried recognizes the particular difficulties of adjusting to a rather reserved and xenophobic society. Fried describes the Swedish educational facilities organized specifically to support child survivors in the absence of family. Café 84, one such facility that came into being decades later, continues to be a gathering place for the now-aging survivors who remained in Sweden. It is a place to socialize and, with the help of a psychologist (individually or in groups), to confront painful memories as well as current crises. The diary of a young survivor enlivens this account.

History of the Australian Child Survivor Groups includes reports from a Melbourne group by Paul Valent and the Sydney group by Litzi Hart. This chapter describes the events and people instrumental in organizing these informal yet extremely cohesive, effective, and viable groups. Personal trauma were processed, and the healing power of relationships among people with a common background is affirmed in the context of a stable group.

While the experiences of German children during World War II are comparable neither to the horrors lived through by Jewish children in hiding and in concentration camps, nor to the children in occupied countries, some German children nonetheless suffered trauma. The chapter, Trauma: A View from the German Side, is based on the life stories of East and West Germans, told during interviews conducted before and after the 1989 unification. Charlotte Kahn discusses their manner of coping, adult lives, attitudes toward family and political life, and their reflections on childhood experiences of evacuation, relocation, bombings, hunger, fear, and incarceration. At the time of the unification of East and West Germany—a time of great political, ideological, and economic upheaval—the trauma of youth was reawakened in some older Germans.

My Contra-Program: A Response to My Father is an autobiographical account by Gonda Scheffel-Baars, the daughter of a Dutch Nazi. She reveals the physical and psychological suffering of being victimized in her own home, the hurt of being a pariah in her community, the burdens of a life-long series of ailments, and finally the satisfaction of attaining inner harmony with the help of religious faith, a sympathetic counselor, and an understanding husband. Like many other collaborators' and Nazis' children, the author unconsciously developed a "program" opposite to that of her father.

Although the interests and activities of that program were born out of resistance, their intrinsic content ultimately engaged her, and emancipated her from resistance to her parents. Now she takes pride in being a teacher of adults in need of a "second chance."

NOTES

1. See "Introduction," this volume.

2. Henry Krystal, "Trauma and Affects," in *The Psychoanalytic Study of the Child*, 53 vols. (New Haven, Conn.: Yale University Press, 1978), 33:81–116, quote cited on 97.

3. See "Introduction," this volume.

4. Anna Freud, *The Ego and The Mechanisms of Defence*, trans. Cecil Baines (1936; New York: International Universities Press, 1946).

5. Judith S. Kestenberg, "Children Who Survived the Holocaust," *International Journal of Psychoanalysis* 67, no. 3 (1986): 309–316, quote cited on 310.

6. H. Dasberg, "Psychological Distress of Holocaust Survivors and Offspring in Israel," *Israel Journal of Psychiatry and Related Sciences* 24 (1987): 243–56.

7. Gertrude Blanck and Rubin Blanck, *Ego Psychology: Theory and Practice* (New York: Columbia University Press, 1974), 93.

8. Lybda Share, *If Someone Speaks, It Gets Lighter* (Hillsdale, N.J.: Analytic Press, 1994), 117, 127.

9. Peter Shabad, "Repetition and Incomplete Mourning: The Intergenerational Transmission of Traumatic Themes," *Psychoanalytic Psychology* 10, no. 1 (1993): 61.

10. See "Introduction," this volume.

8

Child Survivors: A Review

Paul Valent

Introduction

Why were child survivors rediscovered only after a latent period of forty years? Could there be a parallel in the current rediscovery of sexual abuse of children, which Freud pointed out almost a century ago?[1] Today, we have become aware of the extent to which children are exposed to violence, rape, and the witnessing of violent death.[2] It may be that these childhood traumas are reflected adult vulnerabilities. Ambivalent to children, such adults can pass traumatic experiences on to them.

Until recent times, children were treated as chattel and slaves, dehumanized of personality and sensitivity. Especially in times of scarcity, the drain they imposed was limited by low fertility, contraception, abortion or infanticide, and even cannibalism.[3] Some scholars speculate that the Nazis displaced the impulses to loot, dehumanize, and even cannibalize their own children onto Jewish children.[4]

Child survivors of the Holocaust are a fertile group for the study of effects of childhood trauma. The specific traumas and their contexts are well documented—as are the concurrent traumas of parents—and the survivors' progress has been observed over a period of half a century.[5] At the time of the Holocaust, children underwent possibly the greatest attack in history on every aspect of their existence. They were the most vulnerable group marked for the most extreme extinction by the most powerful dictatorship. Nine-tenths of Jewish children in Nazi Europe were killed. Further, these children came from a culture known to highly value family life and children. A study of the psychological impact of the Holocaust on child survivors can illuminate the lifetime effects of childhood trauma in general.

HISTORY

Though definitions vary, in this chapter, a child survivor is any Jewish child who survived in Nazi-occupied Europe, by whatever means, and who was not older than sixteen at the end of World War II.[6]

The psychosocial sequelae of the Holocaust were recognized in adults in the 1960s, and in the 1970s attention was focused on the children of these adult survivors.[7] Except for Polish and rare English literature in the immediate postwar years, child survivors were recognized only in the 1980s—that is after a period of forty years or more.[8]

Krell noted that even child survivors did not recognize themselves in this interim period.[9] They demurred, saying that their parents were the real survivors, they were "only children" in the war and that they had no memories. This perceived lack of impact of the war because of youth contrasts with clinical observations that the younger the survivor, the greater were the potential harmful effects of traumatic experiences.[10] As with adult survivors, early studies of child survivors tended to be pessimistic. For instance, over half of the psychiatrically hospitalized child survivors were noted to be psychotic, the proportion being greater in younger survivors.[11] However, in nonclinical samples, the proportion of psychiatric illness was much smaller. In particular, Moskovitz and Hemmendinger, who respectively followed up on children from orphanages in England and France thirty years later, were impressed with the resilience and high degree of socialization of these child survivors, even though some of them had needed psychiatric help.[12]

At present, the literature on child survivors has expanded. Two journals have devoted special sections to them.[13] Child survivors themselves have experienced a parallel subjective awakening, shown by the 1,600 who rallied to meet in New York in May 1991 at The Hidden Child Conference. Articles and books on child survivors have proliferated since then.

WARTIME TRAUMATIC SITUATIONS

Child survivors were not spared any of the horrors of the systematic methods to extirpate Jews forever.[14] Their inability to work hard, to execute orders, and the requirements arising from their immaturity were treated with special impatience and brutality. For instance, infants who could not evacuate a hospital in Lodz ghetto during a roundup were thrown out of the window. Killing and such heinous acts as using infants for target practice, medical experimentation and castration, and burning and torturing them were legally sanctioned.[15]

Children also had to share their parents' segregation, overcrowding, starvation, cold, humiliation, and the wearing of the yellow star. Some children survived by hiding, and all children were potential victims of roundups, mass shootings, and deportations in jammed cattle trucks. In concentration camps, if fit enough, they had to perform slave labor. Among many other horrors, they endured forced marches.

Mitigating these circumstances for children was adult protection. On the other hand, parental disappearance, total parental helplessness, and death were constant, real threats. Traumatic events occurred fast. A knock on the door in the middle of the night, and helpless parents were taken away forever. Parents suddenly gave children away to strangers. Separation from parents, for a period of time at least, was almost ubiquitous. Even when they did not witness brutality and death, fears of such events were transmitted to the children.

Some substitute caretakers were loving. However, even constant parent substitutes often disciplined the children by threatening to turn them over to the authorities, and fully one-sixth of a sample of hidden children had been sexually molested.[16] Hiding with a series of unsympathetic caretakers could be more distressing than a concentration camp.[17] Abandonment, hostile adults, and annihilation were a constant potential reality for many.

Lack of regularity, sequence, and constancy, including the interruption of school and play, constituted interferences in children's developmental phases and normal growth.[18]

ACUTE RESPONSES

As long as the parental protective shield and faith in parental omnipotence persisted, children were cushioned somewhat against objective horrors and deaths, and they could afford to interpret external events partly in terms of their developmental level and tasks.[19] For example, humiliation for being Jews could be experienced in terms of adolescent peer rejection, or deportation perceived as an adventure.[20]

Older children who had to assume adult roles and children whose protective shield was impaired, experienced dread, fear, desolation, torment, and death in the manner of adults.[21] Operating simultaneously was a psychological imperative to experience traumatic events from their viewpoint as children. For instance, a survivor explained that while hiding, "there was always a devil, in the figure of death who would catch me. When I saw the dead person physically (in concentration camp), I was less afraid than when I felt the fear of being taken [by the devil]. . . ."[22]

Verbally and nonverbally, adults imparted the dread of death to the children with great clarity and used this dread to extract extreme obedience and adjustments, especially in times of extreme danger. Thus children could be made to hide in small spaces for long periods, sometimes on their own; to keep quiet for an inordinate time; and to assume a series of false identities, even while separated from parents. Adult-like affects were countered with adult-like defenses. For instance, instead of sobs at losing a whole family, a twelve year old felt a tearing loose in the chest, and "The small childish sobs did not come, instead my chest felt crushed with the mature agony of an entire people."[23] As in adults, traumatic events were accompanied by mental numbness and a sense of unreality.[24] This included an intense freezing of feelings. Expression of terror, grief, despair, pain, anger, and guilt could have compromised the child's life. Surprisingly, children as young as four could take correct actions, such as hiding under the sheets or running to a neighbor.[25]

A capacity to not feel and to become apathetic (even to death) helped children to survive the traumas of parental helplessness and loss, and to face murder, torture, and death.[26] Two other psychic adjustments helped survival: an inner drive felt as a compulsion to live and a tenacious secret clinging to a good object, ultimately representing loving parents. Such bridging objects could be tangible, as, for instance, lockets or combs, or the last intangible words of parents, "Remember your (shot) brother." "Survive for us." Intangible fragments of memories and feeling states could also be cherished and preserved through various symbolic substitutes.[27] Sometimes the symbolic substitutes were real people who sacrificed heroically for the children, who might have experienced their rescuers as nameless disappearing objects, perhaps linked by fragments of goodness. The younger the child, the more difficult it was to remember such "good objects."

Fear and dread were the constant background to continued denial or numbing. At times, though, subacute events (such as a religious father ordering the family to eat pork, or the child's learning of his doctor's suicide) could release the emotions and a sense of the world in utter turmoil.[28]

Two factors contributed to the children's reactions: their developmental stages and their reliance on parents. Control over their psyches was tenuous for children up to the ages of three or four. Their worlds could fragment, and they could neither understand nor contain their emotions.[29] Sometimes they responded somatically, perhaps with asthma or diarrhea, or with inappropriate behavior.[30] They were the group most dangerous to rescuers. Six year olds, too, especially when away from knowing adults, could falter with their rote-learnt identities and give themselves away. But even very young children could understand what was going on. For instance, a three year old told an SS man that he should not kill her as she had good hands for work.[31]

Children's traumatic events were experienced in terms of connections to parents and caretakers. Core traumatic moments in concentration camps were those of separations and deaths of parents and relatives. The "last looks," especially, and the last things said were remembered forever.[32] While events were appraised realistically, they were also imbued with childlike hopes, judgments, and meanings—such as separations being judged as abandonments evoking anger or self-blame and guilt. One self-critical child said, "I chose to stay in bed while my parents were led away."[33]

Total parental powerlessness and vulnerability were irreconcilable with the struggle for life. Therefore, even while emotions, negative judgments, and meanings were frozen, an adaptive, internal representation of psychosocial relations had to be preserved for the fight for life to continue. For the parents, children were not only the center of the struggles for survival, but also a source of danger and a burden to highly strained adults. Though negative emotions and acts were more frequently expressed by substitute caretakers, at times parents confronted the tragic dilemma presented in the novel and film *Sophie's Choice*: the forced abandonments of children to their certain death.[34] Parents, too, froze the emotions, guilt, and meanings of these traumatic situations.

Despite the inhuman circumstances, children never quite lost their creativeness and age-appropriate fantasies. Children engaged in excited, though somewhat muted, play around destroyed buildings, as would children in normal circumstances.[35] Play was present wherever it was possible, in ghettos and even concentration camps where children played at death games.

The innocence and hopes expressed in children's games were precious to adults, who dared not hope so openly. Even *SS* guards could be moved by such games.[36] Curiosity survived, too. Dori Laub described how he wondered, "What is father thinking?" as they plodded through the snow.[37] He asked a man what he was thinking after a public flogging in a concentration camp. The curious boy became a social scientist.

A striking agreement on the children's reactions is recorded in the literature. To the extent remembered, events seem vivid, constant over the years, and valid when tested.

LIBERATION AND POSTWAR RESPONSES

The most hardened Allied soldiers were moved to tears when they saw concentration camp child survivors. For the children themselves, liberation was both a "joyous running, falling, feeling the fear, then getting up to run again," and a beginning understanding of the enormity of what had happened: "Suddenly, I saw that I had no one . . . absolutely nothing."[38] Some died of overeating and many took ill after liberation. One child survivor suggested that many overate in order to die because despair overtook them.[39] One way to cope was to continue the survival mentality of not feeling, simply plodding forward to the future.

Postwar stresses could be as severe for some as those of wartime. Some needed to recognize that families were lost forever. Some had to separate from loving caretakers and return to biological parents who had become strangers. Even when they were remembered, parents had changed or had new partners. Parents who could no longer cope, or those needing recuperation, placed their children into orphanages—a bitter betrayal of wartime hopes. Other children returned to hostile, antisemitic environments. For those who emigrated, their past lives became unreal as adoptive parents and adoptive countrymen seemed indifferent to the survivors' sufferings and wanted them to discard the past.

In the weeks and months following liberation, habits acquired during incarceration or hiding persisted. Children released from camps appeared greedy for food, quarreled to get it, tended to be undisciplined, and lacked social skills. They experienced numerous childhood neurotic symptoms such as bed wetting, clinging, poor sleep, nightmares, and an inability to trust adults and others. However, most children eventually responded to care, became socialized, and formed friendships.[40]

Psychologically, child survivors coped with additional postwar traumatic situations on the one hand by repressing past memories and feelings, and treating remaining memories as belonging to an irrelevant past; and, on the other hand, by dealing with current stresses as they did with past ones, that is, by cutting off the present and focusing on the future.[41]

BUILDING AND REBUILDING LIVES (LATENT PERIOD)

Child survivors continued to isolate and encapsulate the past while laboring hard to establish security. Many became financially successful, married, and became devoted parents. Many joined the helping professions and were otherwise worthwhile and even altruistic members of society.[42] As there was wonder at the end of the war that these children had survived, there was wonder now at how well they had done.[43] Even so, some became psychotic, while others displayed a variety of posttraumatic stress responses, including nightmares, physical symptoms, emotional states, and disjointed memories that often made no sense.[44] Perhaps most continued silently to yearn to belong, to have fuller, loving relationships, and to enjoy the world with humor and optimism.[45]

It is too easy to take one or another position about the ability of child survivors to build normal lives. In fact, there seems to be a mixture of spirit of survival—which carried the children beyond their earlier suffering—with the Holocaust's continuous, penetrating influence over their lives. For instance, one of the survivors with a normal, jovial appearance and a "good" outcome wrote of a chronic, dominant, pervasive feeling related to his mother, whom he could not remember: "I feel lost, waiting to be found."[46]

Child survivors who grew up with their survivor parents shared some of the problems of second-generation children. Parental anxiety over their survival often led to close but problematic relationships, and in some families the children were seen in terms of killed and potentially dead children. At the same time, they were to support their distressed parents, bear testimony, and accomplish dreams of being "well." In turn, child survivors could become parents who imposed similar burdens on their own children, but with less access to the knowledge of what they were doing.[47]

Perhaps the dilemma of wellness—clouded by concurrent, pervasive, bur-

densome, and undefined feelings—may be explained by the lack of or suppression of memories. Child survivors were told that they could not
remember, should not remember, and what they remembered was invalid.
"Since you were only a child and can't remember, it didn't mean anything."[48] Kestenberg noted that memories may not come to consciousness
if either the parents or the superego opposes their emergence.[49] This was
legally sanctioned in German restitution laws.[50] Child survivors continued
to arrange their psyches according to environmental demands.

However, not remembering also continued to be the key defense against
the pain of traumas. It came to be aided by other psychological defenses—
negation, denial, and repression.[51] Isolation of affect and depriving the event
of meaning, significance, and true knowledge allowed for "half-knowing."[52]
Neither child survivors nor their parents wanted to expose to each other the
frozen judgments and meanings of their pasts. They shared a "conspiracy
of silence."[53] Child survivors were often drawn to each other in their teens
without knowing why. They did not share their Holocaust secrets with each
other, either. The silence was shared by peers and outsiders, too.

This phase seems to have encompassed a long latency period during which
child survivors were forgotten and seemed to have forgotten about themselves.[54] Only after more than twenty-five years had elapsed did child survivors begin to think actively about the Holocaust and to reconnect with
their experiences; after thirty-five to forty-five years they began to identify
themselves as child survivors.[55]

CHILD SURVIVORS NOW

Child survivors are now in their fifties and sixties. Perhaps they needed
the perspective of age, the security of rebuilt lives, children and grandchildren of their own, and the waning influence of their parents to reconsider
their traumas and to replace the frozen meanings of their traumas with new
meanings in their lives.

In order to reevaluate their experiences, child survivors need to retrieve
their memories, come into touch with the emotions surrounding their core
traumatic experiences and generally come to terms with their identities.[56]
While some child survivors balk at these challenges, and to variable degrees
continue in their survivor modes, these issues are of major concern to most
of them today.

Identity

The need to accept the identity of a child survivor is contrary to the
previous survival need to hide one's Jewishness. Acceptance requires over-
coming shame for being identified with a degraded, inferior, persecuted
people; adult survivor discounting; and the fear of being excluded (in some

countries) from jobs and homes that constitute a normal life.[57] Such fears are still valid in some Eastern European countries[58] where it may be more difficult to face the persecutors' contempt, general indifference, and the stigma of being damaged or abnormal.

For some child survivors, clear identification as a Jewish survivor may produce conflicts around loyalty to caring Christian rescuers and the Christian religion, which they had come to accept.[59]

On the other hand, accepting the identity of child survivor allows membership in child survivor groups and the realization that one is neither alone nor inferior. Emotional connections with history and with one's own past family—usually ordinary and loving human beings—may be re-established. A view of oneself as having been a victim and now being a survivor may engender pride rather than rejection, and give rise to a sense of being a special witness who can contribute to the prevention of similar crimes.

Integrating Memories and Trauma

Integrating one's life requires a confrontation with the memories of what was survived as a child. Many survivors experience a hunger for memories as if life depended on it, because without memories, the sense of loss of an important part of oneself prevails.[60] "Memories make us feel alive, and as we connect them to the present and the future, we triumph over death."[61] Memories can be fleshed out by reading, talking to others (especially the older survivors) and visiting the places of wartime experiences. Some survivors write of their experiences to make sure they are not forgotten in the future.

To remember, one must break the conspiracy of silence and overcome the fear that this "might unleash the demons of remembrance to haunt the already haunted."[62] Yet even when memories are retrieved, they are associated with the numbing, dissociation, splitting, and the double world of the child in the traumatic situation.[63] It is only when there is full permission to explore the personal judgments and meanings frozen within the situations that memories may have their full emotional impact and allow true integration.

This means that the demons of remembrance include not only terrifying experiences, but also intensely painful interpersonal feelings. According to Kestenberg, anger at abandoning parents is the greatest, yet least worked through problem in child survivors.[64] Survivor guilt and shame, especially difficult to bear when relatives had perished, were often at the core of blocked mourning.[65] Thawing of these emotions can lead to release of anger and assertiveness, sadness and crying, mourning and repair of relationships.[66]

Meanings, Values, Purpose

It has been difficult to extract positive meanings from the Holocaust. Negative meanings came easily, such as parental helplessness or the constant possibility of abandonment to a cruel fate.[67] There was a clash between Jewish values of concern, humanism, and charity, and the mistrust and selfishness generated to survive. Values were shaken. The very fact of parents' survival could evoke suspicions that they did so through promiscuity and immorality.[68]

Holocaust experiences negated the most basic sense of natural justice and emphasized ultimate perversions of law and order.[69] That the world stood by and allowed the wholesale murder of children and their families led to a cynical view of an unjust world. It seemed well-nigh impossible to reconcile a moral Jewish God and the Holocaust.

And yet each child was the carrier of good meanings as none would have survived without care—a scarce commodity that could have cost the lives of the rescuers and caretakers. Thus, as well as being "ultimate victims," child survivors were also especially valuable "ultimate survivors." When the special caretaker was perceived of as God, survival could be seen as a special miracle for God's special purpose. This view allowed a personal reconnection to religion.[70]

More broadly, survival itself was imbued with the meaning of having defeated Hitler's plan.[71] Being the last direct witnesses to the ultimate evil, survivors hope that their special significance in bearing witness and giving testimony may build a bridge between the dead and the thread of one's life in the world, thereby averting similar evil in the future.[72]

CHILD SURVIVORS AND THE FUTURE

Children of child survivors represent defeat of genocide in perpetuity. Child survivors invest passionately in their children's survival and security. While wanting their children to be free of their own sufferings, they also want them to continue to bear testimony to the Holocaust. The offspring of child survivors seem to sense their parents' contradictory desires, just as child survivors perceived those of their own parents.

As a group, child survivors have grown up to be empathic, compassionate with the deprived, and sensitive to injustice, especially when inflicted on the weak.[73] These qualities have made them prominent in the helping professions and in the field of morals. Based on their experiences, child survivors also have produced many works of art and science, and recently, there has been a surge in studies and writings on their parents and themselves.

Helping Child Survivors

Experiences wherein child survivors learn to validate their identities without shame, to retrieve memories, and to find their life-purpose have been found to be helpful. Krell noted that documentary testimonies of child survivor experiences are positive because they help to remember, elucidate, and give chronology to past events, and they confirm, give recognition, and provide meaning for the future.[74] Child survivor groups provide a sense of belonging. They help validate memories and identities, and they provide a forum to share as well as to enjoy.[75] Fogelman noted that group therapy and intergenerational groups can facilitate mourning and release new energy.[76] Little has been written on individual therapy, though many child survivors have sought it and it is probably the only way to deal with some traumas. Moskovitz and Krell pointed to the importance of sympathetic recognition to overcome survivors' shame.[77] Kestenberg described a technique of bringing back memories by helping the survivor "imagine" within a supportive relationship.[78] But most important, it is essential to be aware of the existence of child survivors and their traumas and of one's own tendency to feel numb and unable to listen to their stories.[79] Otherwise, even long contact with them may miss the point of their problems.

DISCUSSION

Child survivors of the Holocaust offer an unprecedented opportunity to study the effects of childhood trauma over the life cycle. Knowledge of their traumatic situations, as well as prospective and retrospective studies, all indicate that child survivors' traumas had marked effects on them throughout their lives, a phenomenon also documented for soldiers and concentration-camp survivors and, long before that, put forward by Breuer and Freud.[80][81][82] Major long-term effects have also been documented prospectively in individual patients, but not previously for a large group.[83] Unlike the questions of validity of childhood memories surrounding sexual traumas, there is no question that the child survivor's traumas actually occurred.

At the time, the children dealt with their concurrent perceptions, emotions, judgments, and meanings of the crumbling of their external and internal worlds by dissociation from the event. They "froze" their reactions into numbness and were determined to live to make up for the present in the future. Doing otherwise would have threatened survival. The "culture" of these responses was determined by the stage of development of the child and the traumatic situations. Core traumatic Holocaust situations were more complex, and therefore could potentially be more overwhelming to the child's ego than particular traumatic excitations (as in sexual abuse, for example). However, even in the Holocaust situation, the ego was not globally overwhelmed, having constricted instead to meet survival needs.[84]

This initial complexity was increased by subsequent stresses and traumas in wartime and after, akin to concepts of "cumulative trauma."[85] Survivors reached variable equilibria of reliving and avoiding the components of their traumas, and the traumas variably pervaded their personalities and existential outlooks. This view extends Freud's and is in line with traditional views as well as those of modern theorists.[86]

Symptoms could vary greatly, aspects of the traumatic situation being represented somatically, in action, or psychologically. However, even when well defended and relatively symptom free, individuals were intensely affected. Perhaps the invisible pervasiveness of Holocaust trauma is like a saturated solution on the verge of crystallization. The solution looks normal, but much internal energy is devoted to making it seem so. Kestenberg called this a tension "beyond diagnosis."[87] This state could cause as much distraction from enjoyment of life as symptoms and illnesses (crystallizations from the solution). As noted also in other traumatized groups, the latent post-Holocaust period of rebuilding was the outward manifestation of making life as normal as possible.

Regarding previous vulnerability as a determinant to later responses, it must first be acknowledged that for many children there was hardly a "previous time." The literature implies that subsequent distress responses nevertheless formed quite uniform constellations, with variations predominantly influenced by the number, severity, and type of traumas. This resembles the findings for adult Holocaust survivors and for combat soldiers.[88]

Child survivors seem to share features with other traumatized groups. They share with the adult "survivor syndrome" sequelae of anxiety, disturbances in cognition and memory, a tendency toward isolation, inability to verbalize the traumatic events, unresolved mourning, guilt, and rage against parents who failed to protect them.[89] They share with the children of survivors a parental overprotection and fear of the environment, separation problems, taking on parental missions, shame, and "feeling different" from the normal population while appearing to be successful (often in helping professions).[90] Their responses have similarities to other war child survivors and with child survivors of nonwar traumas, such as childhood abuse and incest.[91] Traumatized groups show much similarity in their trauma responses, though each has its own specific features. For instance, child survivors tend not to be aggressive, possibly because in their traumatic situations aggression would have meant death.

CONCLUSION

One-and-a-half million children were purposefully murdered in the Holocaust. The children who survived underwent major, well-documented traumas. These child survivors are a valuable source for the study of trauma. Indeed, they present a unique opportunity to learn about the long-term effects of trauma on children.

This chapter has detailed some of the trauma-induced responses. Many questions about the nature of trauma and its associations with perceptions, emotions, judgments, meaning, and moral issues require further exploration. Similarly, the complex nature of trauma responses and the complexity that child survivors present, as well as the overlap of the child-survivor experience with the traumas of other groups, should alert us to the importance of an expanded theory of trauma and its effects.

The needs of many recently traumatized children in so many quarters of the world and the newer waves of child survivors from countries of persecution remind us that childhood trauma is common and should always be considered in our patients and in our students. Child survivors of the Holocaust give us hope that even the most vulnerable victims of the greatest of traumas can have their humanity and dignity restored.

NOTES

1. Sigmund Freud, "The Aetiology of Hysteria" (1896), in *The Standard Edition of the Complete Psychological Works of Sigmund Freud* (London: The Hogarth Press, 1962), 3:191–221.

2. Robert S. Pynoos and Kathy Nader, "Children's Exposure to Violence," *Psychiatric Annals* 20 (1990): 334–44.

3. Richard Lee and Irven DeVore, *Man the Hunter* (Chicago: Aldine, 1977), 11; Geza Roheim, *Psychoanalysis and Anthropology* (New York: International Universities Press, 1968), 150.

4. Judith S. Kestenberg and Janet Kestenberg-Amighi, "The Jewish Quest for Life and the Nazis' Quest for Death," in *The Psychological Perspective of the Holocaust and Its Aftermath*, ed. Randolph L. Braham (Boulder, Colo.: Social Science Monograph; New York: Csengeri Institute for Holocaust Studies, Graduate School University Center of the City University of New York, distributed by Columbia University Press, 1988), 13–44.

5. Deborah Dwork, *Children with a Star* (New Haven: Yale University Press, 1991).

6. Robert Krell, "Therapeutic Value of Documenting Child Survivors," *Journal of the American Academy of Child Psychiatry* 24 (1985): 397–400.

7. Henry Krystal and William Niederland, "Clinical Observations on the Survivor Syndrome," in *Massive Psychic Trauma*, ed. Henry Krystal (New York: International Universities Press, 1968); and Martin S. Bergmann and Milton E. Jucovy, *Generations of the Holocaust* (New York: Basic Books, 1982).

8. Anna Freud and Sophie Dann, "An Experiment in Group Upbringing," in *The Psychoanalytic Study of the Child*, 53 vols. (New York: International Universities Press, 1951), 6:127–68; Sarah Moskovitz, *Love Despite Hate* (New York: Schocken Books, 1983); Judith S. Kestenberg and Milton Kestenberg, "The Sense of Belonging and Altruism in Children Who Survived the Holocaust," *Psychoanalytic Review* 75 (1988): 533–60.

9. Robert Krell, "Therapeutic Value"; Robert Krell, "Child Survivors of the Holocaust Forty Years Later," *Journal of the American Academy of Child Psychiatry* 24 (1985): 378–80.

10. Judith S. Kestenberg and Ira Brenner, "Children Who Survived the Holocaust: The Role of Rules and Routines in the Development of the Superego," *International Journal of Psychoanalysis* 67 (1986): 309–19.

11. Krell, "Child Survivors."

12. Moskovitz, *Love*; J. Hemmendinger, *Survivors: Children of the Holocaust* (New York: National Press, 1986).

13. "Child Survivors of the Holocaust," *The Journal of the American Academy of Child Psychiatry* 24, no. 4 (1985):377–40. *The Psychoanalytic Review*, 75 (1988).

14. Dwork, *Children with a Star.*

15. Milton Kestenberg, "Legal Aspects of Child Persecution During the Holocaust," *Journal of the American Academy of Child Psychiatry* 24 (1985):381–84.

16. Sarah Moskovitz and Robert Krell, "Child Survivors of the Holocaust: Psychological Adaptations to Survival," *Israel Journal of Psychiatry and Related Sciences*, 27 (1990):81–91.

17. Kestenberg and Brenner, "Children Who Survived."

18. Ibid.

19. L. Rotenberg, "A Child Survivor/Psychiatrists's Personal Adaptation," *Journal of the American Academy of Child Psychiatry* 24 (1985):385–89.

20. Theresa I. Cahn, "The Diary of an Adolescent Girl in the Ghetto: A Study of Age-specific Reactions to the Holocaust," *Psychoanalytic Review* 75 (1988):589–617.

21. Moskovitz and Krell, "Psychological Adaptations."

22. Yolanda Gampel, "Facing War, Murder, Torture, and Death in Latency," *Psychoanalytic Review* 75 (1988):506.

23. Kestenberg and Brenner, "Children Who Survived," 311.

24. Flora Hogman, "Roles of Memory in Lives of World War II Orphans," *Journal of the American Academy of Child Psychiatry* 24 (1985):390–96.

25. Ibid.

26. Gampel, "Facing War."

27. Ira Brenner, "Multisensory Bridges in Response to Object Loss During the Holocaust," *Psychoanalytic Review* 75 (1988): 573–87.

28. Rotenberg, "Survivor/Psychiatrist."

29. Judith S. Kestenberg, "The Response of the Child to the Rescuer," presentation at the Faith in Humankind Conference. Unpublished Manuscript, 1984.

30. Kestenberg and Brenner, "Children Who Survived."

31. Judith Kestenberg, personal communication, 1990.

32. Hogman, "Roles of Memory" Brenner, "Multisensory Bridges."

33. Hogman, ibid., 394.

34. Sarah Moskovitz, "Barriers to Gratitude," in *Remembering for the Future* (Oxford: Permagon Press, 1988); William Styron, *Sophie's Choice* (London: Cape Press, 1979); Paul Valent, "The Psychological Impact of Being a Hidden Child," presentation at The Hidden Child Conference, New York, 1991.

35. Gampel, "Facing War."

36. George Eisen, *Children at Play in the Holocaust* (Amherst: University of Massachusetts Press, 1988).

37. Dori Laub, "Auschwitz at 16 and at 61," presentation at the Conference Society for Traumatic Stress Studies, 1989.

38. Moskovitz and Krell, "Psychological Adaptations," 83; Gampel, "Facing War," 508.

39. Paul Valent, "Effects of the Holocaust on Child Survivors," *Australian and New Zealand Association of Psychotherapy Bulletin* 1 (1990): 12–16.

40. Freud and Dann, "Group Upbringing"; Moskovitz, *Love*; Hemmendinger, *Survivors*.

41. A. Mazur et al., "Holocaust Survivors: Coping with Post-traumatic Memories in Childhood and 40 Years Later," *Journal of Traumatic Stress* 3 (1990):1–14.

42. Kestenberg and Kestenberg, "Sense of Belonging."

43. Moskovitz, *Love*; Hemmendinger, *Survivors*.

44. Krell, "Child Survivors."

45. Gampel, "Facing War"; Rotenberg, "Survivor/Psychiatrist."

46. Moskovitz, *Love*, 403.

47. Valent, "Psychological Impact."

48. Moskovitz, *Love*, 402.

49. Judith S. Kestenberg, "Imagining and Remembering," *Israel Journal of Psychiatry and Related Science* 24(1987): 229–31.

50. M. Kestenberg, "Legal Aspects."

51. Mazur et al., "Holocaust Survivors."

52. Kestenberg, "Imagining."

53. Peter Sichrovsky, *Strangers in Their Own Land* (London: I. B. Tauris, 1986).

54. Mazur et al., "Holocaust Survivors."

55. Rotenberg, "Survivor/Psychiatrist."

56. Valent, "Effects."

57. Moskovitz, *Love*.

58. Kestenberg and Kestenberg, "Sense of Belonging."

59. Flora Hogman, "The Experience of Catholicism for Jewish Children During World War II," *Psychoanalytic Review* 75 (1988): 511–32.

60. Judith S. Kestenberg, "Memories from Early Childhood," *Psychoanalytic Review* 75 (1988): 561–71.

61. Kestenberg, "Memories," 571.

62. Krell, "Therapeutic Value," 400.

63. Kestenberg, "Memories"; Dori Laub, "Knowing and Not Knowing Massive Psychic Trauma: Forms of Traumatic Memory," presentation at the Conference Society for Traumatic Stress Studies, 1989.

64. Judith S. Kestenberg, personal communication, 1990.

65. Moskovitz and Krell, "Psychological Adaptations."

66. Mazur et al., "Holocaust Survivors"; Kestenberg and Brenner, "Children Who Survived."

67. Valent, "Effects."

68. Eva Fogelman, "Intergenerational Group Therapy: Child Survivors of the Holocaust and Offspring of Survivors," *Psychoanalytic Review*, 75, no. 4 (1988): 619–40.

69. M. Kestenberg, "Legal Aspects."

70. Fogelman, "Intergenerational."

71. Kestenberg and Kestenberg, "Sense of Belonging."

72. Ibid.

73. Moskovitz, *Love*; M. Kestenberg, "Legal Aspects"; Kestenberg and Kestenberg, "Sense of Belonging."

74. Krell, "Therapeutic Value."

75. Kestenberg and Kestenberg, "Sense of Belonging."

76. Fogelman, "Intergenerational" Eva Fogelman, "Group Treatment as a Therapeutic Modality for Generations of the Holocaust," in *Healing Their Wounds: Psychotherapy with Holocaust Survivors and Their Families*, ed. Paul Marcus and Alan Rosenberg (New York: Praeger, 1989).

77. Moskovitz and Krell, "Psychological Adaptations."

78. Kestenberg, "Imagining."

79. Krell, "Child Survivors."

80. Dwork, *Star*; Moskovitz, *Love*; Hemmendinger, *Survivors*.

81. H. Klonoff, G. McDougall, C. Clark, et al., "The Neuropsychological, Psychiatric, and Physical Effects of Prolonged and Severe Stress: 30 Years Later," *Journal of Nervous and Mental Disease* 163 (1976): 246–52; Krystal and Niederland, "Clinical Observations."

82. Joseph Breuer and Sigmund Freud, "On the Psychical Mechanism of Hysterical Phenomena: A Preliminary Communication" (1893), *Standard Edition* (1955), 2: 3–17.

83. Albert J. Solnit and Ernst Kris, "Trauma and Infantile Experiences: A Longitudinal Perspective," in *Psychic Trauma*, ed. S. S. Fürst (New York: Basic Books, 1967), 175–224.

84. Freud, *"Inhibitions, Symptoms and Anxiety"* (1926), *Standard Edition* (1959), 20:87–156.

85. Masud R. Khan, "Ego Distortion, Cumulative Trauma, and the Role of Reconstruction in the Analytic Situation," *International Journal of Psychoanalysis* 45 (1964):272–79.

86. Freud, *"Moses and Monotheism"* (1939), *Standard Edition* (1964), 23:7–137; B. A. Van der Kolk, ed., *Psychological Trauma* (Washington, D.C.: American Psychiatric Press, 1987).

87. Judith S. Kestenberg, personal communication, 1990.

88. Fred Hocking, "Human Reactions to Extreme Environmental Stress," *Medical Journal of Austin* 2 (1965): 477–83.

89. Krystal and Niederland, "Clinical Observations."

90. Arlene Steinberg, "Holocaust Survivors and Their Children: A Review of the Literature," in *Healing Their Wounds: Psychotherapy with Holocaust Survivors and Their Families*, ed. Paul Marcus and Alan Rosenberg (New York: Praeger, 1989).

91. Dorothy Burlingham and Anna Freud, *Young Children in Wartime* (London: George Allen and Unwin, 1942); Morris Fraser, *Children in Conflict* (London: Secker and Warburg, 1973); Mary Donaldson and Russell Gardner, "Diagnosis and Treatment of Traumatic Stress among Women after Childhood Incest," in *Trauma and Its Wake*, ed. Charles R. Figley (New York: Brunner Mazel, 1985).

9

Nazi Fathers

Judith S. Kestenberg

INTRODUCTION

The general consensus among many students of Nazi behavior is that Nazis were able to be cruel to Jews and their other victims while being kind and loving fathers to their own children.[1] Lifton labels this process "doubling."[2]

Juelich, a German psychoanalyst, questions this, holding that the portrait of the *SS* man or soldier as good husband and father is a cliché. Juelich notes that Nazi propaganda appeared to favor the family, but in reality destroyed it.[3] He offers data from his analysis of second-generation Germans, particularly children of Nazis, to support his position. For example, one patient was put under such great pressure by his Nazi father that he thought he had no right to live, but must sacrifice his life for the Fatherland.

Juelich suggests that Nazi families coped with the discordance in their lives not by forgetting and repressing (as is suggested by Mitscherlich and Mitscherlich), but rather by the defensive process of "splitting."[4] Nazi fathers split off their guilt about murder and torture of victims and projected it onto others, primarily the Jews. Did the use of splitting permit some men to be kind fathers?

Rottgardt has discussed the use of silence, probably the most common defense used in the postwar period.[5] Nazi parents refused to discuss the atrocities with their children, building a wall around themselves. Their children, in identification with them, refused to acknowledge what their parents had done.[6] Bar-On calls this barrier between them a "double wall."[7] Were there effective barriers or defenses that permitted a man to be cruel in one context and loving in another? If not, what were the ways in which the two seemingly separate worlds of family life and Nazi murder were interconnected and yet held apart?

Although interview data do not give us the kind of depth of insight found in analytic material, studying a number of published interviews and some of our own interviews of children of Nazis or collaborators enabled us to survey a larger number of cases, discover various patterns, and compare and contrast them to theories presented in the literature.[8]

In this chapter I hope to show ways in which the cruel behavior engendered by Nazi goals affected patterns of fathering by many Nazis and collaborators. Likewise I hypothesize that Germanic traditions encouraged hostile feelings toward their children, which were at times projected outward, making atrocities against children of Jews and Gypsies, as well as other weak and defenseless people, emotionally more acceptable. Finally, where Nazi fathers have been described as being loving, I will attempt to show the psychological processes that may have made it possible for them to act this way.

INTERVIEWEES SPEAK OF THEIR FATHERS

In a survey of interviews, I found that about 41 percent of the adult children of Nazis described their fathers as cruel, authoritarian, and distant.[9] In the remaining interviews some described their fathers as kind, loving, and playful with their children; and a larger number did not discuss their relationships with their fathers at all.

One of the most common themes found among both kind, loving fathers and cruel, authoritarian ones was that of not seeing, not speaking, and not knowing. This kept knowledge of atrocities away from the family, but also impeded communication within the family. During and after the war, Nazi fathers either pretended not to know anything about the crimes toward humanity, or they said that they were helpless bystanders. In short, they did not acknowledge the effects of their actions or inaction.

It was not that they always had to obey orders or were helpless observers. Protest and resistance by German citizens was often effective, particularly in the early years. For example, when the Nazis decreed that Nazi re-education would replace religious education, the parents in one German province got together and protested. As a result, the order was rescinded. Although individual protest was often dangerous, group protests were effective.

Because people did not look when Jewish children were taken out of school, did not see when neighbors were arrested or taken off to concentration camps, they could claim that they had no ability to stop the carnage. German people had no difficulty describing their army experiences, but responded to the topic of the murder of innocent people by saying either, "We also suffered," or by claiming that during war regular laws don't hold up.[10] Some, particularly the members of the Weimar youth generation, spoke of World War II only in terms of the battlefields. They did not talk of their Nazi past, only of the war. To them the army was beyond reproach. They fought a war, nothing else; they did not know about the shooting of

Russian prisoners. Only a few were guilt-ridden. Amongst these was one so tortured by the memory of his deeds that he needed psychiatric help and hospitalization. Many more defended themselves by denying the atrocities. Hans Pfeiffer compared the bombing of German cities and their civilians to the genocide perpetrated by the war criminals, and suggested that, consequently, England and America should have gone on trial at Nuremberg as well.[11] He claims that the German people did not know, but repeatedly acknowledges their looking away and forgetting. This denial rendered them silent and uncommunicative, not only as citizens of postwar Germany, but also as fathers.

Silent Fathers: Mrs. V. A. and Mrs. N. M.

Mrs. V. A. was born in 1941 in Heidelberg. Her father volunteered for the *SS* in 1943. He prided himself on being a good soldier, but after the war he could not get a job because he had been a Party member. He bore it staunchly. He would not bend. Even when his daughter reached out a helping hand to him, he would not take it. He isolated himself from the family and eventually became an alcoholic.

His daughter was tortured by the question, why had her father joined the *Waffen SS*? Surely he must have believed in Hitler. Even if she couldn't understand him, he still was her father, and she had a special bond with him. Although he fought with her mother and hit her brother, her tears could always get him to stop. When she grew up she became a music therapist, working with alcoholics (like her father); it was she who found an old-age home for her father. But even she described him as being "like a stone." Until death, he was a silent old man.

Many others tried to approach their parents to find out what happened during the Nazi era, but usually they were silenced. Speaking of the Holocaust, Mrs. N. M.'s father said, "One has to leave it alone, in peace." Hearing this, she said, made her throat constrict. In another case, a daughter tells of feeling close to her father, recognizing his shortcomings and loving him still, but being unable to reach him. She knew he was a difficult person—often unhappy, often angry—which she tried to excuse by pointing to his difficult childhood and the severe beatings by his own father. But there were many times when they did not talk to each other. The silence stood like a wall of stone commemorating the dead, she said.

An Ambivalent Father: Mr. X. H.

In a few cases, rather than silence there was conflict within the father between knowing and not knowing, telling and not telling, caring and not caring. X. H.'s father was authoritarian and often cruel, but clearly ambivalent about many things. He adored Hitler, yet often criticized him.

He perceived the war years as a suspension of reality, and hoped it would eventually usher in a new era.

Coming from a patriotic German family, X. H.'s father joined the army serving in southern Russia, France, and Poland. Like many others, he said that he had done nothing wrong. He couldn't have done such things and did not want to hear or talk about it. However, he reproached himself for never having taken any action, saying, "I could have known, but simply didn't believe it was so bad." When people were throwing a piano out of a house during *Kristallnacht* (Night of Broken Glass), X. H.'s father became enraged. On the other hand, he did not allow his family to listen to a foreign radio station. When the older brother was not promoted in the army, X. H.'s father said that Hitler was a criminal, but later he said that if Hitler knew about the corruption going on, he would clean things up after the war.

X. H. himself identified with his father and followed a similar program of openness and denial. In 1942, when he was fourteen, he witnessed concentration-camp inmates who were forced to clean up after the bombing. They were emaciated. He talked to a classmate about it, wanting to hear a denial. Instead, the anti-Nazi classmate told him of relatives in concentration camps. "It was depressing and I put it out of my mind," X. H. said.[12] [13]

Vindictive and Neglectful Fathers: Miss J. T.

In quite a number of interviews, adult children described vindictive and cruel fathers who beat their children, flew into rages, hit their wives, and did not allow their views to be questioned. For example, Miss J. T., born in Stuttgart in 1948, spoke of her father as a sadistic man who had vicious temper tantrums. Only as a teenager did she have the courage to ask him his opinion about the Holocaust. His answer was, "I don't like the Jews anyway." She did not dare ask whether he meant that it was acceptable, therefore, to exterminate them. She concluded that he knew of the fate of the Jews and chose not speak about them. Despite his cruelty and prejudice, she felt a strong bond with her father, albeit one that became increasingly disturbed as she matured and questioned the past. She was not insulated from her father's Nazi experiences.

Many children were abandoned by their fathers, as was a Norwegian woman who recently wrote to me about her childhood. Her father had promised to return home after the war, but never did. For a time, her brother was placed in a children's home close to her father, who occasionally visited him. However, neither she nor her brother ever saw their father being loving or responsible. On the contrary, she was frightened of him, and noted in her letter that the Norwegian word for father, *faren*, is the same as the word for *danger*. She wrote that her father was too bad to be true, and her mother was too good to be true.

In many cases the cruelty and the emotional distance led to painful feelings of rejection. Several interviewees spoke of feeling like stepchildren or orphans in the family. Some parents were so involved in the Nazi cause, they had no time for their children. Fathers went off to the army or wartime jobs, and mothers often attended meetings. Home life often resembled a boot camp. Many parents assigned heavy chores to their children. One interviewee's father threatened to throw her out of the house if she didn't do her chores, as though she had betrayed her family. This father had beaten his wife and then, when she fell ill, transferred his aggressive impulses to his children. His daughter described him as unable to experience his own feelings, a man so dedicated to Nazi goals, so caught up in the national trauma of Germany, so identified with Hitler, that he suggested that the whole family commit suicide when Hitler died. Their lives were held to be of little account.

CHILDREN AS VICTIMS

Abused Child: J. H.

Often, as J. H.'s situation illustrates, the maltreatment of the children had implicit or explicit parallels to the treatment of Jews and other Holocaust victims. J. H. was born in 1930 in Hamburg. His parents did not allow him to play with Jewish children, though they did not speak of the persecution of Jews in the home. J. H. knew something of it from newspaper accounts; however, it seemed distant from his life. J. H.'s mother frequently beat him with the metal part of a belt, and his father was not only strict but unduly demanding. As a small child, J. H. already had to work long hours in the house and garden. When a new baby was born into the family his father told him that his mother will "no longer have time for him. You must help more." When his baby sister had diarrhea, J. H. had to sleep on a mat in front of her bed. He felt like vomiting, but had to obey nonetheless.

Leaving home, whether to the Hitler Youth or with his school group, was a relief to him, even when he was sent away with his school class for nine months to a new place where life was difficult. It was freezing and snowy, his parents had sent along only short pants, and he was traumatized by the harsh rules of the camp. But for him the worst thing was the sight of so many Jewish transport people begging for water. When one man put his arm out to reach for the water, someone shot his arm off. Though the sight disturbed him, he did not condemn the treatment of the Jews.

While other children cried with homesickness, J. H. felt only relief and wondered whether he had no feelings for his family. His father sent back his letters with spelling corrections rather than sympathy for his plight. J. H. vowed never to treat his children so badly. Though a victim of his parents' stoicism and ideology, he never identified himself with other Nazi victims who suffered aggression. They occupied worlds apart.

Sick Child

In some cases, there was a more open ambivalence about the intrusion of the Nazi world into the home. S. H. was born in 1940, in Berlin. Among her first comments during her interview were, "My father was a Nazi," and "I've made peace with my parents."

Because S. H. was born with a tumor, her paternal grandfather, a Protestant clergyman, refused to baptize her. She remembers her mother telling her many times how ugly she was. She was "too fat, had crooked legs, and a tumor." In 1945 she was sent to a hospital to have an operation. She feared being killed there, especially upon seeing other children who had been burnt by sulfur. When she tried to get up to help them, the nurses tied her to the bed, where she remained alone until after her operation. When ready to leave the hospital, she was sent to live with her grandfather, and even when she finally returned home, her mother was always busy, often away.

Ironically, the house in which she was born and raised had been taken from a Jewish family. In this formerly Jewish house now lived people with a strong Nazi ideology. S. H. remembers the joyful reception of a package in her house containing the book *Mein Kampf*. Her parents dreamed of the "Final Victory." Though in 1952 they had been forced out of "their" house and left with nothing, her parents continued to celebrate Hitler's birthday. Because they celebrated an ideology that condemned the "handicapped" to inferiority and possible extermination, the parents were ashamed of their daughter.

After the war, S. H. found herself both seeking peace with her parents and accusing them—not of mistreating her, but of adhering to Nazi ideology. Her father would not respond to her, at once pretending to be hard of hearing and claiming she had been "indoctrinated" by the lessons now taught at school. Talking to him was like "talking to a concrete wall." Finally, much to her father's dismay, she planned a trip to Israel. Was she seeking to punish him? Was she seeking out other victims? When invited to be interviewed, she initially refused to talk to a Jewish interviewer, but then agreed to come, indicating her conflict between identifying with her parents on the one hand and with the victims (a category of people from whom she was able to escape) on the other.

Children Identify with Victim and Perpetrator: Mrs. Stegmann

Researchers have often encountered children of perpetrators who identified with the Jews.[14] Hardtmann long ago referred to her children-of-Nazis analysands as the "Jews of their parents," which means to me that they were persecuted by their parents.[15] Bar-On interviewed fifty-one children of perpetrators and witnesses of the Holocaust, located through advertisements and personal connections.[16] Among them was Mrs. Stegmann (a pseudonym), who described herself in an interview as a victim of her parents, especially her father, who had been actively involved in the euthanasia program of the Nazis. Mrs. Stegmann's parents were members of the Nazi Party since 1932. In 1933 her father, a doctor, became head of a district department of health. His job was to dismiss Jewish physicians, sterilize forced-labor women, and advise physicians in his district about the selection of patients for euthanasia and the transportation of children to Hadamar, an institution where mentally ill and retarded children were gassed.

Mrs. Stegmann had one surviving brother. (Another brother with a club foot had died as an infant.) Her parents had forbidden the children to use the entrance to the house that her father's patients used, for fear of contamination. One day when she was four years old, she attempted to enter that way nevertheless, and when her brother tried to prevent her, she smashed a window in anger. Her father gave her such a spanking that she had to stay in bed for days, and from then on, she was afraid of her father. Now she blames her mother for not protecting her.

She claims that in the Third Reich boys were more valued than girls and that she had not been a wanted child. During the bombings, she was seized with panic and screamed with fear in the air-raid shelter. Father rushed to hold the shelter door shut, but never took her on his lap, which left her feeling rejected by him. Her mother was not particularly warm either. Returning from a sojourn on a farm, her mother, instead of embracing her, began checking her hair for lice. Mrs. Stegmann reposts that while her mother was examining her, she felt frightened for her life. Did she identify with disheveled Jews and mental patients she may have seen, or perhaps even with the lice?

Though some of Mrs. Stegmann's stories showed her parents as loving, in her summation of her own case, she emphasized their general lack of love and stated, "My parents were cruel and did not love me."

There is considerable evidence that she made an unconscious connection between her own suffering and the suffering of her father's victims. She was frightened by the delousing experience, by her infant brother's death, and by the death of unknown children. When she and her brother accidentally discovered their dead brother's grave, her mother reacted with such fury that the children asked no more questions. Her mother did not seem sad (presumably because the child had had a club foot and was handicapped.) Mrs. Stegmann herself was near-sighted, but as a child she hid this from her parents. She explained that she wanted to be able to see "so that she could live." Not until after the war, when she no longer feared her father, did she admit to her near-sightedness. But even then the bed she slept in as a child haunted her because their building had formerly been used to house mentally ill children, many of whom had been sent to Hadamar by her father. For years she had recurrent nightmares about this.

When her younger brother was a baby, her father, wanting to test whether his son was fit to live because he looked so Jewish, threw him into the swimming pool. The child was saved by an older sister.[17] Bar-On and Rosenthal believe that she perceived her family to be a threat to her right to life and suggest that she pseudoidentified with the victims of the Nazis.[18] (It is not clear to me why they use the term "pseudo." Perhaps they are reluctant to see this as a pure identification because she was also identified with her parents in many ways.) As in other cases described above, she was a victim of her parents' hostility and the Nazi ideology. Nevertheless, until 1945, Mrs. Stegmann considered herself a Nazi follower, an admirer of Hitler, and proud to be the daughter of high-ranking Nazi parents. She cried for hours upon hearing of Hitler's death and felt, "My world collapsed at that point." Bar-On and Rosenthal rightly state that identifying herself as a victim of her parents may have helped allay her guilt feelings about her Nazism. Her sense of being in danger early in childhood and her identification as her father's victim fused with both his aggression toward her and her discovery of more and more of her father's atrocities.

As an adult, she was not freed from these feelings. Her father was sentenced to five years of hard labor, but returned to private practice after his release in 1949. He died in 1957. If she required a stronger punishment to expiate the guilt further, it came to her in the form of her mother's cancer and death, followed by her son's death from leukemia shortly thereafter. Bar-On and Rosenthal wonder whether she might in some way consider these deaths a punishment.[19]

The Disgraced Child of a Collaborator: G. S.-B.

The last case in this section is that of Gonda Scheffel-Baars, born in Holland in 1942. She has written her story, the story of a Dutch collaborator's daughter who suffers during the post-war period on account of her father's deeds.[20] For reasons she does not know, her father hated Jews and supported the occupiers in their aims to annihilate the Jewish people. But her troubles stemmed not only from the family's social disgrace (accruing from father's collaboration with the Nazis), but from her father's sexism. While he was happy about having a son, like all patriarchal fathers, he was disappointed that her brother was not like him, but weak and asthmatic—not at all like father. On the other hand, she had more of the qualities a father expected in a son, but she was a girl and the father was not one to accept people the way they were. He was subject to occasional temper tantrums, particularly against women. She felt like an orphan in her parental house, a child fallen from heaven into some strange house. About her father's behavior during the war she had heard little, but asks, "My father killed me with his words and behavior, so what worse had I to hear?"

Worse was her persecution by the community for her father's misdeeds, from which she came to hear more about his wartime activities. Her brother had a breakdown when he heard about his father's past and was unable to finish high school. She recalls, "The first time I wanted to kill myself was when I was eighteen" while waiting alone at a train station, thinking that desperate people jump in front of trains. "I could not sleep that night," she reports, and the other nights of the week were a horror. This nightmare and the feelings of horror returned recurrently, driving her to seek relief in religion. She says "I found my hold in life in my faith. My history studies revealed that the roots of Christianity were found in Judaism and so I began to learn Hebrew and Jewish ideas were good enough to build my life with. Like many collaborator's children, I developed a counter-program to the life's program of my father, of course, unconsciously."

Interestingly, G. S.-B., though she does not feel fully loved by her father, has much compassion for him and identifies with him in some ways. She also feels rejected by him personally, as well as by his deeds, which she tries to negate. Negating him, of whom she is part, leads to a wish for self-negation (which she was later to overcome with the help of a clergyman and a psychotherapist).

CONNECTIONS BETWEEN FATHERS' TREATMENT OF THEIR CHILDREN AND NAZI VICTIMS

Nazi Ideology

All of the fathers discussed above were to some extent cruel and despotic toward both their own children and the victims of the Nazis. As small children, and later as adults recalling the past, the children suffered at their fathers' hands. Although these fathers' behavior toward Nazi victims and toward their own children clearly differed, it seems warranted to say that there was a connection. I hypothesize that Nazi ideology negatively affected paternal behavior. For example, children who had serious imperfections were mistreated and perhaps even killed. Harshness toward children, long a German tradition, was intensified. Although parents did not often speak to children about their SS work or collaboration, children nevertheless frequently identified with the victims of their father's actions. Parents' aggressive behavior took on much stronger implications within the destructive setting of Nazi Germany, where even children were victimized. Several fathers stated that they disliked Jews, as if this were sufficient cause for them to be killed. Similarly, many of these children felt as though their parents disliked them. Did this make them vulnerable to persecution as well? Of course, portraying themselves as their fathers' victims, adult children are offering themselves up as a way to reduce the guilt they feel for their fathers' acts. Nevertheless, in my view the children did not "pseudoidentify," but truly identified with Nazi victims. This came about as a result of their fathers' application of Nazi ideology and Nazi practices to some aspects of the paternal role.

Death Wishes Toward Their Own Children

I further hypothesize that Nazi parents had an unconscious wish to kill their own children, a wish projected onto the Jews, Gypsies, handicapped, homosexuals, and others who were adversaries of the Nazi government. Nazis accused Jews of obscure plans to govern the world and characterized them as enemies of Germany, referring to them as vermin, which, according to Freud, is a symbol for small children. To protect themselves against the Jews (unconsciously the representatives of their own unruly children), Nazis rendered adult victims helpless by starving and working them to death.[21]

We can see evidence of German aggressive feelings toward their children in the suffering of little children in fairy tales such as Hänsel and Gretl. We also see it in harsh and emotionally distant paternal parenting, which was not only common at the time, but also the ideal, meant to produce strong, resilient sons. It is particularly evident in fathers who knowingly and purposely exposed their children to acts of cruelty against others, which, like the fairy tales, suggest punishments that might befall the child, too, if it doesn't please its parents.

For example, Amon Goeth, the Nazi leader of Plaszow, taught his four-year-old son how to play "pigeons" by throwing Jewish infants up in the air and shooting them. Schwammberger, who ruled the camps of eastern Poland in a most cruel way, brought his four-year-old son along when he forced a Jew to undress and then playfully shot him. The child laughed.[22]

HOME AND ENVIRONMENT ARE MUTUALLY REINFORCING

It becomes evident, then, that the Nazi environment encouraged hostile behavior toward its own children, and that, in turn, encouraged implementation of the Nazi design. Thus, the general environment and the home environment in Germany often exerted a mutually reinforcing force. Hitler Youth taught young people to disdain the weak and turn on them, a behavior supported by their experiences at home at the hands of abusive and emotionally distant parents. It was a fatal combination, leading neighbors and friends to behave in ways that few expected and no one predicted.

Although the brutal Nazi father who victimized his own children (as well as Jews) was common enough to be well represented in most collections of interviews, it was not the exclusive pattern among Nazis. Some children of Nazis recall fathers who spent long hours playing with them, fathers portrayed as being loving and kind. Though they often added that their fathers sometimes had temper tantrums, these were erratic and not the dominant theme of their relationship to their children. This is the kind of situation Lifton labeled as a case of doubling, and Juelich considers to be a result of the "splitting" process.

Splitting and Child-like Behavior: Mr. A. T.

The case of Mr. A. T. might explain this pattern of splitting. He was born in Heidelberg, in 1925. His mother was a strict Catholic, and his father was in the *SS*. A. T.'s father led transports of Jews, and A. T. often saw Poles and Jews being transferred out. At that time though, "one didn't think anything of it." When his father came home on furlough, he used to play "army" with the children, who were second lieutenants and had to "show their nails and teeth." In 1944, the father was assigned to Buchenwald, where his son visited him. It is interesting that this "kind" father exposed his son to his "work" environment. A. T. claims there were no Germans there—only Russians, Hungarians and French, all in uniform. (This is obviously mistaken information. There were many Germans there, not to speak of A. T.'s father himself.) In 1950, A. T.'s father was sent home, apparently after a long de-Nazification program. Nevertheless the children were proud of their father. They had participated in the war, via play and some exposure, and upheld their father's role in it.

With the mother, the situation was different. A. T. praised her for engaging in various charitable acts, such as giving bread to columns of prisoners as they marched by and cooking food for the Russians, hiding these deeds from her husband. However A. T. also praised his father for good deeds and qualities, bragging that he was the best prisoner, who gave his bread to younger soldiers. "He was more manly, harder than I," A. T. explained. In sum, he portrays his father as a good man; his mother as an angel.

When asked whether he had investigated his father's activities during the war, he answered, "I would never do it. [Then] I could not have respect for him and I could not love him. You should have seen how he played with us. He could whirl us in the air; he pulled and carried us around. . . . Even when we were ten years old, he pulled us around on sleds. . . . I love him very much. He was like a child. I don't want to know about it. It would hurt him and it would break my heart." Actually, A. T. often disguised his father's misdeeds, for example, by misrepresenting his father's de-Nazification as a prisoner-of-war internment.

This is a typical case of a father who acted like a child with his children, and they loved him for it. Nevertheless, he was not the man his son wanted him to be. Perhaps contrasting the two parents, saying that his father was good and his mother an angel, was a vaguely implied criticism of the father. A. T. denied the truth because, as he admitted, it would break his heart to think badly of his father or to hurt him. He spoke about his father with a compassion, tolerance, and pride one usually reserves for children. One cannot stay angry at a child for its misbehavior when most of the time it is fun-loving and kind.

From this case and others similar to it, it appears that there was a group of men who regressed or never matured who were great playmates with their children, but erratic fathers. They did not teach a system of ethics to their children, who, if they learned one from their mothers, had trouble applying it to their fathers. They, after all, were only children—children like themselves, easily led into committing terrible acts, without straining their consciences. The child-like fathers did not have to separate their home lives and behavior from their public lives because in each they believed they were simply following the rules and doing as they were told. Angry and aggressive at times, they were usually forgiven because, as one woman said, "when father was joking around, he was irresistible." I suggest, therefore, that regression to an immature mentality, or an insufficient development to a mature mentality, played an important role in producing what appears to be discordant behavior. Their childlike quality tied together their apparently discrepant behavior.

GENERATIONAL TRANSMISSION OF BRUTALITY

Children's Obligation to Confirm Father's Ideal

Despite the variety of parenting styles among Nazi fathers and collaborators, hostile behavior appears to be common. These behaviors should be seen as products of the Nazi environment, which required more loyalty to the fatherland than to the family and encouraged aggression towards the weak. They were also the product of aggressive attitudes toward children within the domestic sphere. Many of these aggressive fathers were themselves raised by brutal fathers and raised their own children accordingly. They punished children who did not meet the ideal of a child who contributes to the father's good image and becomes a perfect extension of father's ideal self. Ideal children do not drain away father's energy and resources.

Of course, no child can meet these ideals, and, at times, all parents feel ambivalent toward their children. But the cultural setting in Germany fostered the authoritarian, intolerant, and often cruel father and husband.

Like children, Jews had been taken in by Germany and given a homeland there, but were not obedient and humble in that they maintained some trappings of their own identity and treated their children differently from the Germans. When not perceived as competitors, Jews were seen (like children) as imposing an economic drain on Germany. Thus, Jews representing children who have to be destroyed, cleaned from the womb so that Germany could undergo a rebirth, were particularly suitable victims.[23]

CONCLUSION

Summary

It appears that, in most cases, the enemy without was often confused and intermixed with the enemy within. In only a few cases was any real separation effected between the world of atrocities and the world of the home—even the playful Nazi father brought his son with him to "work." Moreover, the common use of silence as a defense could not stem all knowledge or remove from the family the aura of cruelty and hostility that permeated all life under the Nazis.

Thus, weak and imperfect German children were mistreated as well, while those who were more able to conform to parental ideals—the perfect lambs—were sent to Hitler Youth camps and to the war, sacrificed so that the nation might live. If the war had not ended when it did, would the "loving" father who played "army" with his son have sent him willingly to die for his country? That would have been the logical culmination of the war games.

It is important to collect more such cases and attend to a variety of experiences and behaviors. Nazi mothers, for example, need to be studied more thoroughly from the psychological point of view.[24] It appears that while many of them were cruel also, they were often deeply religious and thus more inclined to help than were the fathers.[25] It is also important to hear the stories and understand the motives of those who resisted and those who attempted to save the victims. But that is another study.[26]

Significance for Understanding Child Abuse

Our findings on Nazi fathers have great significance for an understanding of the effects of child abuse in American culture. It is well known that abused children are more apt to become abusive parents. Our material suggests that they are also more apt to abuse many others who are unable to protect themselves. We know, for instance, that Hitler's father beat his dog until he crawled under the table and wet himself. He abused his son Alois, and when Alois ran away at fourteen, his wrath was turned on Adolf.[27] Stangl had a similar history.[28] His mother enjoined Stangl's father to stop beating him because the child's blood was spattering on a freshly painted wall. There was no sympathy at home for Hitler or Stangl. Hitler, of course, was full of rage and became paranoid. He felt compelled not only to exterminate the Jews, but to send the youth of Germany to their deaths. Even as he glorified the youngsters, he taught them to die bravely for the fatherland, and sent twelve to sixteen year olds to war at the last minute, knowing full well they could not win against their stronger adversaries.

The abuse suffered by children becomes a model for their future ways of relating to others. Their identification with the aggressive parent as well as the child victim renders them both aggressive and fearful. Two cult leaders, David Koresh and Jim Jones, were men neglected by their fathers who projected their childhood fears into fears of the outside world. Ultimately, this lead them to a self-destruction paralleling Hitler's own death.[29] The patriarchal father, German or American, creates a model for violence that a charismatic leader can direct into feelings of hatred and deeds of torment against any scapegoats.

Thus, it seems that abusive American fathers might also have become Nazis had they been given encouragement from a government such as the Third Reich. There is danger everywhere.

NOTES

1. Robert J. Lifton, *The Nazi Doctors* (New York: Basic Books, 1986).

2. Ibid.

3. Dierk Juelich, *Geschichte als Trauma* (Frankfurt: Nexus Verlag, 1991); and idem, "Experienced and Inherited Trauma," Presentation at the National Israeli Center for Psychosocial Support of Survivors of the Holocaust and the Second Generation (AMCHA), Israel, May 11, 1993.

4. Alexander Mitscherlich and Margarete Mitscherlich, *The Inability to Mourn* (Munich: R. Piper, 1967).

5. Elke Rottgardt, *Elternhörigkeit: Nationalsozialismus in der Generation danach. Eltern-Kind-Verhältnisse vor dem Hintergrund der nationalsozialistischen Vergangenheit* (Parent-dependence: National socialism in the next generation. Parent-child relationships in the context of the national-socialist past) (Hamburg: Verlag Dr. Kovac, 1993).

6. Ibid.

7. Dan Bar-On, *Legacy of Silence: Encounters with Children of the Third Reich* (Cambridge: Harvard University Press, 1989).

8. I am grateful to the students of Professor Hannes Friedrich, to Dr. Gertrud Hardtmann, and to Dr. Peter Brundl and his group for the interviews, which in addition to my own, helped to provide the data for this paper.

9. This figure is based on thirteen out of forty interviews of my own, fourteen interviews conducted by Bar-On (1989), thirteen interviews by von Westernhagen (1987), and fourteen interviews by Peter Sichrovsky, *Born Guilty: Children of Nazi Families* (New York: Basic Books, 1988). Of these forty-seven, thirty-three spoke openly of aggressive fathers, while the remainder either said little about their fathers, did not know their fathers, or in a very few cases, spoke of loving fathers.

10. Gabriele Rosenthal, ed., "Als der Krieg kam, hatte ich mit Hitler nichts mehr zu tun" (When the war came, I had no business with Hitler anymore), in *Zur Gegenwärtigkeit des Dritten Reiches in Erzählten Lebensgeschichten* (On the presence of the Third Reich in narrated life stories) (Opladen: Leske & Budrich, 1990).

11. Hans Pfeiffer, *Sagen wie es war* (To say it as it was) (Krefeld: Sinus Verlag, 1988).

12. The not hearing, ignoring, and holding in oblivion is the system used by two year olds who do not want to stop playing when called away from a game.

13. Gertrud Hardtmann, "Von unerträglicher Schuld zu erträglichem Schuldgefühl" (From unbearable guilt into bearable guilt feelings), in *Der Holocaust: Familiale und Gesellschaftliche Folgen* (The Holocaust: Familial and societal consequences), ed. Dan Bar-On, F. Beiner, and Manfred Brusten (Wuppertal, Germany: University of Wuppertal, 1988), 56–61.

14. Gabriele Rosenthal and Dan Bar-On, "A Biographical Case Study of a Victimizer's Daughter's Strategy: Pseudo-Identification with the Victims of the Holocaust," *Journal of Narrative and Life History* 2, no. 2 (1992): 105–27.

15. Gertrud Hardtmann, "The Shadows of the Past," in *Generations of the Holocaust*, ed. Martin S. Bergmann and Milton E. Jucovy (New York: Basic Books, 1982), 228–44.

16. Bar-On, *Legacy of Silence.*

17. Gabriele Rosenthal, personal communication, 1994.

18. Bar-On and Rosenthal, "Biographical Case Study."

19. Ibid.

20. See Chapter 17, this volume.

21. Judith S. Kestenberg and Janet Kestenberg-Amighi, "The Jewish Quest for life and the Nazis' Quest for Death," in *The Psychological Perspective of the Holocaust and Its Aftermath*, ed. Randolph L. Braham (Boulder, Colo.: Social Science Monograph; New York: Csengeri Institute for Holocaust Studies, Graduate School University Center of the City University of New York, distributed by Columbia University Press, 1988), 13–44.

22. Aaron Freiwald and Martin Mendelsohn, *The Last Nazi* (New York: W. W. Norton, 1994). For further evidence supporting this view see our earlier article, Kestenberg and Kestenberg-Amighi, "The Jewish Quest for Life."

23. Magdalene Schultz, "The Blood Libel: A Motif in the History of Childhood," *The Journal of Psychohistory* 14, no. 1 (1986): 1–24. Some Germans were particularly angered and resentful of the ways in which Jewish and Gypsy children were "spoiled" by their parents. Perhaps this spoiling of children was a cause of jealousy. As Schultz has suggested, because Jews love their children so, the Nazis put the blame for child killing on them. Jews were accused of drinking the blood of gentile children, and one interviewee was told that there was not enough milk for her, and she would stay small because of the Jews.

24. Claudia Koonz, *Mothers in the Fatherland* (New York: St. Martin's Press, 1987).

25. Alison Owings, *Frauen: German Women Recall the Third Reich* (New Brunswick, N.J.: Rutgers University Press, 1994).

26. See Eva Fogelman, *Conscience and Courage* (New York: Anchor Books, Doubleday, 1994).

27. Charles B. Flood, *Hitler: The Path to Power* (Boston: Houghton Mifflin, 1989).

28. Gitta Sereny, *Into That Darkness* (New York: Vintage Books, 1983).

29. P. A. Olsson, "In Search of their Fathers-Themselves: Jim Jones and David Koresh," *Mind and Human Interaction* 5, no. 3 (1994): 86–96.

10

The Persecution of Polish Children

Judith S. Kestenberg

INTRODUCTION

Polish or German, Jewish or Christian, the physical organisms of young children are alike in their vulnerability, and their incomplete personality structures are similarly delicate. However, their life circumstances vary in the available supports and opportunities, or undermining deficits and obstacles. This chapter discusses some of these similarities and differences as seen through a young Polish child's World War II experiences. Although the early damage to her significantly crippled her emotional and physical health, she managed to achieve vocationally and to structure an apparently normal life for herself. That this paradoxical manifestation is almost paradigmatic for childhood trauma survivors becomes evident from the almost ubiquitous appearance of this phenomenon in survivor-interview protocols.

Germans Classify Polish Children

While Jews, Gypsies, and "worthless" German children were subject to extermination, children of Slavs, especially Poles, were divided into three categories: Those whose parents or who themselves participated in the resistance or in the uprising were the so-called "bandits"; those who were taught to become slaves of the Germanic *Herrenrasse*, the "master race"; and those who, due to their Aryan racial characteristics, could be incorporated into the German Reich to become canon fodder for their new country.

In 1944 the majority of the children who were sent to concentration camps—Auschwitz, Gross-Rosen, or Stutthof—were denizens of Warsaw. They either had participated in or endured the uprising against the Germans.

The older Polish children were made to work in camps, where their food was somewhat more plentiful than that of the Jews. The young ones were separated from their parents and placed in children's blocks. For these Polish children, as for the young Jewish victims of oppression whose development through adulthood has been recorded,[1] the consequences of bombardments, devastation, deportation, semistarvation, and separation from their parents were lifelong.

TRAUMATIC MEMORIES

For Polish war victims, the concentration camp experiences are more highlighted than the events preceding them because in Poland former inmates now receive a government subsidy. The frequently occurring separation of mothers and children in camps intensified the already traumatic experiences of deportation and incarceration. The importance of parental support in times of stress and trauma was confirmed by the reactions of British children who endured bombings in the presence of their mothers with fewer negative effects than children who had to tolerate separation from their mothers to be evacuated to safe areas of the country.[2]

Marysia was born in 1941, about two years after the onset of World War II. She was interviewed in Poland in 1989 to tell her story. Among her happy childhood memories was one of being in the company of her mother as she greeted her father on the street when he came home from work and brought her candy.[3] Unfortunately, her happy childhood memories were clouded by subsequent events.

As is often the case for those who were infants at the onset of persecution, Marysia has no memory of German bombardments, hiding in cellars, or marching a long trek, probably carried by her mother to Proszkow near Warsaw, from whence people were deported either to camps or to servitude in Germany. However, subsequent fears of noise may be the body memories of bombs exploding and Germans shouting. Indeed, Marysia reported during her interview that even now she jumps up when a door slams or when someone passes through a corridor adjoining her bedroom at night before she goes to sleep, or when already asleep.

Marysia remembers how scared she was, traveling in the crowded train with her mother on the way to Birkenau (Auschwitz II) in August 1944. Not yet three years old, she clung to her mother for security; then she cried and cried when forcibly separated from her mother to be placed in a children's block. To this day, she is periodically beset by such fears of being alone that she can cope only by asking a co-worker to stay with her overnight.

Most of Marysia's memories of traumatic experiences stand out against a general background of being with many children and going hungry. She doesn't have an absolutely clear picture of all the circumstances, but she is certain of the many children there. She especially recalls the little ones who were around when she was sitting on an upper bunk as a relative came in to give her a potato; he himself ate the peels. She is afraid of hunger, crying, and screaming. During the interview she cried, sobbed, trembled, and had to be calmed before mentioning that she witnessed a dog throwing itself on a small child and tearing it to pieces, This experience left her with a permanent fear of dogs so great that on seeing a dog she must quickly cross the street to avoid it.

She has been told about her frequent illnesses in camp: scarlet fever, measles, pneumonia, and others. To be with Marysia in the hospital, to take care of her and protect her from the multitude of cockroaches, her mother injured her own throat with a needle.

Marysia stayed in camp from the end of August 1944 to the end of January 1945—five months of her young life. She, who had learned to walk at nine months, could no longer walk and had to be carried out of Auschwitz by her mother. But the child's ordeals were not yet over. Somehow she reached Krakow where she and her mother slept in a church full of people. Though she doesn't mention how she got to Warsaw, history tells us that typically there was a long wait for the overcrowded trains. In Warsaw, they saw that their former home had been bombed out. Because Marysia was very sick, mother again took a train to go to her relatives. This was a very stressful period for Marysia and her mother. In vain they waited for Marysia's father until mother heard he had perished in a concentration camp. Mother then became the sole breadwinner of the family, which necessitated leaving Marysia daily. Marysia became shy and distrustful, had difficulties at school, and kept to herself. Nevertheless, she finished business school and found work. Then she attended an evening school to qualify for university studies. Successful in her work, she became a manager. Her subordinates consider her strict but fair and very nervous.

THE AFTERMATH

A late maturer, Marysia did not have a menstrual period until seventeen, which worried both her and her mother. Even though she had expected it, she was very much afraid of it. At twenty, she married and things went well at first. After nine months she bore a son. She was afraid of what would happen to this child, afraid she would transmit to her son her childhood unhappiness of life with her widowed and burdened mother, incapable of sweetness and joy.

In her marriage she was fearful of noises, and her husband could not tolerate her nightly terrors, which woke him. Before long, he began to absent himself from home until finally they divorced. She was left alone with her child and with her mother, who helped her. History repeated itself. She has remained single, rationalizing that no man would tolerate her nervousness. She preferred not to chance another rejection.

Now that her son has married and moved out of town, she is alone again. She receives a government subsidy, but still has to work to make ends meet. Her present illnesses include persecution-related brain damage, evidenced by a disturbed EEG (electroencephalogram); a rheumatic disorder; and a neurosis.

Considering her wartime trauma, personal misfortunes, and her difficulties at school, this victim's professional adjustment is surprisingly excellent. Her combination of disability and excellent performance is characteristic of many other Polish child survivors and may be related to a need for protection and aid and a defense against that vulnerability.

Her fear of noises and of being alone may be understood as a reaction to hiding in cellars when bombing and shooting occurred during the Warsaw uprising, as well as to the separation from her mother in Birkenau. Fear of being alone may also be connected to the recurring experiences of mother and child being left by the husband and father.

Differences Between Jewish and Non-Jewish Polish Survivors

What are the differences between Jewish and Polish survivors? Unlike Jews, Poles after the uprising did not need to fear discovery and betrayal by fellow-Poles, and they did not have to disguise their identity. Poles did not have to fear extermination as the Jews did. Gas chambers were for Jews, not for Poles. There was, however, a camp in close vicinity to the Lodz ghetto designated especially for Polish children of "bandits," about whose imprisonment we have many accounts. For many of the Polish children afflicted with typhus, medical treatment by Jewish doctors constituted their first contact with Jews. Polish children marveled at the kindness of Jewish supervisors sent from the ghetto to supervise their work in the adjoining camp. In contrast, children in camp with some Polish personnel were ordered to throw cold water on a girl who wet herself every night and eventually died as a consequence.

Lebensborn, an institution for pure Aryans, was another terrifying place for Polish children. They were forbidden to speak Polish there and were beaten because they did not know how to speak German. After the war, the Polish commission met with opposition when examining and repatriating these Polish children because they had been placed in pure Nazi families and did not want to return home. Getting 200,000 children of Polish origin back to their country proved to be impossible.

Jewish children who grew up in Poland frequently hid their Jewish identity, and many of them adopted the Catholic religion. One such Catholic child, who was interviewed in her adulthood, had married a Polish poet and bore his child. She remembered that at the age of five, she had accompanied her mother who consulted a lawyer about the case of her daughter. When asked, the mother replied evasively to the effect that the discussion was not about the daughter, but about a namesake. Miraculously, the child believed her. However, during her adolescence, one of her girlfriends at a convent school she attended told her she was Jewish. The mother had disclosed it to one of the nuns, who repeated it to the friend. Upset because her mother had lied to her, the girl ran away from home and hid in her friend's home. After a week her mother came to explain that she had not wanted to hurt the daughter's feelings and they reconciled. She was told the names of relatives in New York, and she wrote and visited them. Nevertheless, she kept her religion and wore a cross on her chest, despite criticism from her grandfather and aunt, who insisted she was a Jewish child.

CHANGED CONDITIONS IN POLAND

After World War II, the Catholic church helped Nazis escape to South America; meanwhile, antisemitism continued to prevail in the Polish villages. Since the end of communist rule, however, the atmosphere in Poland has changed. Jews visit and a resident rabbi teaches Talmud and Torah to those deprived of a Jewish education under communism.[4] Judaism has awakened the interest of the intelligentsia. For instance, a sixteen-year-old young man, informed by his mother that he is Jewish, happily and proudly told his school friends about it. The Association of Child Survivors has 404 Jewish-born members, a surprise considering that only a few people remain who declared themselves Jewish.[5]

The following story depicts the changes since 1989. While visiting the rabbi's educational camp, we met a young boy who asked me to interview his half-Jewish mother, a judge who had two sons by her Polish husband.[6] Even though the country was no longer communist, she feared losing her job because her son had marched in a parade wearing a sweatshirt identifying him as a Jew. This was a problem to her even though non-Jewish Poles who had been incarcerated by the Nazis developed a kinship with the Jews who acknowledge their identity and those who had lived in hiding or had been in concentration camps.

SUMMARY

The experiences of the Polish children, as revealed through interviews and observation, show some of the similarities and differences between the Jewish and non-Jewish children who suffered as a result of the war and the Nazi occupation. The most complex effects, though perhaps not the most serious ones, are manifested by the hidden children whose religious identity was changed.

NOTES

1. Archives of the International Study of Organized Persecution of Children, Tel Aviv University, Tel Aviv, Israel, and Child Development Research, Sands Point, New York.

2. Anna Freud and Dorothy Burlingham, *Infants Without Families* (New York: International Universities Press, 1944).

3. From our archives (interviewed by J. Witkowski). Names are fictitious and personal data have been disguised to preserve anonymity.

4. Ian Buruma, "Poland's *New* Jewish Question," *New York Times Magazine*, August 3, 1997, 34–55.

5. Editor's note [CK]: The number of Poles identifying themselves as Jews is increasing. Elderly parents who had passed as gentiles are telling their children, and people are now able to discover their ancestry in recently financed archives. "Judaism is a new form of chic" with bookstores carrying Judaica and Jewish cafes and restaurants frequented also by non-Jewish Poles. Yet, one mother of a young man interested in learning about Judaism asks, "Who wants to be Jewish in Poland? It can bring nothing but trouble." Buruma, "Poland's *New* Jewish Question."

6. The camp is financed by the Lauder Foundation.

11

Yugoslavian Child Survivors

Nikola Volf

Interviews with adult and child survivors have been conducted from the psychological and psychiatric points of view in many countries. The interview data gleaned from thousands of people is a first-hand documentation of the events that occurred just before, during, and after the Holocaust. Just as important is the evidence that organized oppression does leave psychological traces in the victims of the persecution, but the trauma incurred and the stress endured can be healed to the extent that most of the survivors can lead normal adult lives. At this time, the effects of trauma and the healing process are very important topics especially in light of the current events in this country—which was still Yugoslavia when these interviews were conducted.

This chapter is a brief account of the interviewing project in Yugoslavia: its initiation, process, and results.

INITIATION OF THE PROJECT

About seven years ago, Dr. Judith S. Kestenberg[1] proposed an ambitious plan to conduct a widescale study of the child survivors from all regions of Yugoslavia. Estimating this task as too big for a single researcher, I brought it to the attention of the director of the Institute of Mental Health in Belgrade, a prominent institution with a marked psychosocial approach to psychiatric problems. The institute accepted the project in principle, and I immediately proposed, within the frame of the study, to restrict myself to the Jewish population. Although interest in the planned work abated over time, I remained inclined to perform the study, limiting it to the Jewish community in Yugoslavia, at that time encompassing about 6,000 to 7,000 persons. The Federation for Jewish Communities in Belgrade offered cordial help, in the form of a circular to be sent to all local communities, in order to obtain the names and addresses of all Jews who were thirteen years old and younger at the start of the Holocaust in Yugoslavia. Owing to the shortage of funds and to the distance between the Jewish communities, which were scattered throughout the land, it soon became apparent that my work had to be restricted to a much smaller population. Primarily, I focused on Belgrade (about 1,500 Jews), Subotica and Novi Sad (in the north of Serbia), and Rijeka (Croatia). The large communities of Zagreb and Sarajevo had to be left out, and I had to restrict myself to a total of fifty interviewees.

The following short report is based on some notes made soon after the termination of an interview and on my recollections. All the audiocassettes were sent to Dr. Kestenberg, in New York, to be translated, coded, and interpreted as part of the worldwide study of the organized persecution of children.[2]

As is customary in open-ended, semistructured interviews, I did not in every case stick to the fixed order and to the complete inventory of questions as prescribed in the "guidelines," often leaving the greater part of the interviews to the free communication of the interviewee. My personal evaluations of the interviews are impressionistic because I believe that an exact statistical procedure is not appropriate to a primarily psychodynamically oriented study.[3]

Preliminary contact was often made by telephone, with a short explanation of the aim of this research. The interview itself began with a more detailed explanation of its aims and structure, and usually took place in the interviewee's home. The interviewees signed a consent form, stating their willingness to cooperate freely. They were assured complete anonymity and the right to withhold answers to questions perceived as too personal. With the consent of the interviewee, the dialogue was tape-recorded. Most interviews were conducted in Serbo-Croatian, five in Hungarian, and three in English. The interviews were semistructured, and the dialogue, preparation, discussion, and final comments usually lasted about two hours.

RESULTS OF STUDY

Of the fifty child survivors interviewed, thirty-three were women and seventeen were men, aged mainly fifty to sixty years of age at the time of the interview. There were more Ashkenazi than Sephardic Jews. These proportions reflect the actual gender-ratio and ethnicity of the survivors. A specific feature of Yugoslav history during World War II was the division of Yugoslav territory among several powers (German, Italian, Hungarian, Bulgarian, Albanian, and the Independent Croatian State), a fact reflected in the fate of the local Jewish population. Most of these survivors were confined in concentration camps during the Holocaust, including the most infamous, such as Auschwitz, Jasenovac, Bergen-Belsen, and Theresienstadt. More fortunate survivors were confined in the less brutal camps, as on the island of Rab (under Italian rule). A certain number of Jews succeeded in escaping from the camps to join the Yugoslav partisans where the psychological conditions were far better, although the general conditions were often similar. Child-partisans are a special feature of the Jewish survivors in this country. Often separated from their families, a small number of Jewish children survived by hiding in various, often remote places in Yugoslavia, Hungary, and Albania. Hiding, often requiring a name change and an absolute imperative to conceal one's true identity, resulted in special psychological problems for the child survivor, such as a life-long reluctance to be open about personal matters.

The inconceivable and unprecedented ordeals suffered by camp inmates, especially children, are well known and will not be described here. This short report will address mainly the aftermath of the Holocaust events on the interviewed sample of the population.

Childhood Memories

The majority of the individuals included in this study originated from a liberal religious milieu; the grandparents, not their parents, were the observant Jews, who in some instances played a central emotional role in the life of the children. Kosher food was scarce at that time, and at the time of this study is nonexistent. Yet, childhood memories concerning the atmosphere in the family—the games, Jewish holidays like Purim and Passover, and the special foods connected with them—were often vivid and usually very warmly recollected. Many of these Jewish children were taught to always excel because they are better and cleverer than the other children. However, no interviewee mentioned the clash of such an inner belief with the prevailing realities of their life. Some interviewees declared that under the pressure of Holocaust events, they broke all ties with religious belief, with God, and with their ideals.

LIFE BEFORE THE HOLOCAUST

Relationships with children of other ethnic and religious origins depended much on the prevailing attitudes of the environment. Generally, relations were better with Serbians than with Hungarian and German children. However, in general there were no instances of striking ethnic or religious discrimination toward the interviewees until the beginning of the war, when antisemitic discrimination commenced, largely on the part of the Hungarian and German children.

Although many families tried to conceal the antisemitic events occurring in Europe (mainly in Germany), most children, excepting the very young, knew about the great number of Jewish refugees from Germany and Austria, and intuited these changes, albeit without experiencing outright feelings of fear. Only one woman reported prewar childhood fears, which mainly concerned possible separations from her parents. Her separation fears are very accentuated even now, especially since the beginning of the present civil war in the former Yugoslavia.

The beginning of the war had great impact on the population, as a result of the bombings and the occupation by foreign forces. The antisemitic regulations that ensued added further hardships for Yugoslavian Jews, who were forced (like Jews in all other Nazi-occupied territories) to wear yellow arm bands or stars, interrupt schooling, move to ghettos, and endure separation, deportation, or hiding. These events, combined with "the change of all values" and the humiliation of the parents (mostly the fathers, and often in front of their children), engendered feelings of insecurity, fear, and anxiety. Many interviewees declared that this did not result in the parents' loss of esteem in their (the children's) eyes; indeed, they felt an even greater attachment to their parents.

LIFE DURING THE HOLOCAUST

Instead of enumerating all the unthinkable atrocities that these children endured here, I will confine myself to those events and experiences considered by the survivors to be the worst. These include the physical illnesses that plagued many of the children. They suffered typhoid, malaria, dysentery, pneumonia, furuncles, sores on the head from lice wounds, and swollen feet and joints.

The humiliation and death of their parents were causes of great psychological pain. One set of parents was beaten. One child witnessed the execution of her father; another saw his father dying immediately after listening to Hitler shouting on the radio, even before the Holocaust; still another was separated from the mother in Auschwitz. Even as children, some anticipated their own deaths, as was the experience of the child who had thought he would die without having had his first sexual experience. Another expected to be executed on the shore of the Danube. They also knew that some people died or went mad while being transported in cattle cars.

AFTERMATH OF THE HOLOCAUST

Generally speaking, the largest number of the interviewees were quite sane, without major somatic and psychic pathology, only two of them having had a history of hospitalization in a mental institution. By far, the most common, lasting physical ailments were disturbances of the gastrointestinal system: gastric and duodenal ulcers, periduodenitis, chronic enteritis, and indigestion. To some extent, psychic factors played a role in these disabilities. One interviewee described experiencing difficult situations as if he were ingesting spoiled or poisoned food, saying, "I take all influences through my stomach." Certain other disorders, such as bad teeth and delayed menarche, may be attributed to the poor diet. There were reports of fertility problems requiring long gynecological treatment (which, of course, are harder to trace back to the ghetto and camp conditions of the Holocaust). One woman claimed she stopped growing after living in the concentration camp. The generally unhealthy living conditions, particularly cold and dampness, are associated with chronic rheumatism. Physical wounds remained open a long time after liberation. Both physical and psychological healing proceded slowly.

Fear and anxiety were the most often-mentioned lasting effects of the Holocaust. Irrational fears of hunger and starvation were prominent. For the survivors, bread had truly become the staff of life. They said simply, "My obsession is bread"; "Bread must always be in my home"; "At the end of the meal, I must eat a piece of bread—it is obligatory"; and "I cannot bear bread being thrown away."

Having seen numerous corpses in the camps, many survivors dread going to funerals and fear looking at the dead. They cannot tolerate watching stories about concentration camps on television or in movies, or to see the persecution of Jews or any other people. Generally, media representations of violence and abuse are abhorrent to them. In some persons, the sight of blood also arouses uneasiness.

In some instances, divorce was experienced as a repetition of the forced separation from parents. Brief depressive states were also noted, although some lasted for several months. More severe occurrences of clinical depression were accompanied by suicide attempts. Vague uneasiness, anxiety, insecurity, nervousness, and forgetfulness were also attributed by some interviewees to the aftermath of the Holocaust.

But other, more stoic attitudes also came to light during the interviews. One woman encouraged her younger sister in Auschwitz with the words "We won't cry!" and as a result of this deeply imprinted slogan, she continues to have difficulties crying. Many interviewees described the long search for their lost family members. For many months, daily trips to the railway station ended in deep disappointment when their search proved to be in vain. Still, a psychiatrist declared, "One should never justify one's shortcomings and failures as the consequences of the experiences during the Holocaust; [shortcomings are] a private affair!"[4]

Postliberation nightmares are a common manifestation. Images of Holocaust scenes and wartime experiences often reappear in the survivors' dreams. Germans shouting "*Los, los!*" ("Get moving!" "Shove off!") disturb their sleep. In their dreams, they hide and flee. The nightmares often are unembellished renditions of real events; at other times the memory is represented in a somewhat attenuated edition. Again, separation fear (from parents) haunts them, as in their dreams, they see dead people with the heads of their parents. Another nightmare is of parents' vain attempts to save their children. One writer told the interviewer, "I never dream about camps, but scenes about being escorted to a firing squad, which in reality has never happened; so I dream about a more beautiful, more glorious death!" Some interviewees suffer so much from their dreams that they wake up screaming or are awakened by their spouses.

Under the influence of Yugoslavia's civil war, both nightmares and conscious remembrances of the Holocaust's dreadful events have become more frequent.

ADAPTATION TO THE NEW LIFE AND SURROUNDINGS

Liberation from the oppressors was experienced as an exceptionally joyous event by the majority of survivors, but some of them were so apathetic that it took them several days to become aware of the changes of their fates. The return to their homes took place after many weeks, or even months, of convalescence in special institutions in Germany, Denmark, or Sweden, depending on where the liberation took place. Understandably, upon return to their original milieu, their feelings were largely determined by the presence or absence of their parents, other family members, and their houses.

World Jewish organizations, such as the Joint Distribution Committee and the Federation of Jewish Communities of Yugoslavia, provided great material and moral assistance. The new state, which had fought against the common enemy, also provided some aid. Together, these organizations assisted in finding dwellings and schooling. But the homecoming was frequently embittered by such remarks as, "Look, this bloody Jew managed to come back!" In other instances, the refreshing renewal of old, friendly ties contributed much to the internal, psychic rehabilitation of the survivors. In general, they enjoyed full acceptance by a sympathetic people who, during the war, had themselves been persecuted by the same oppressor, although to a far lesser degree than had been the Jews.

THE HOLOCAUST AS A PIVOTAL POINT IN THE LIFE COURSE

Most of the interviewees considered the life events of the Holocaust a turning point in their lives, declaring that their lives would otherwise have taken a smoother course. Perhaps they could have attained higher achievements in school and career. Only a few of them felt that their "inner" life, their feelings and fantasy life, had become broken: "I would have grown up with a greater sense of security," or "I would have looked at life and endured it more easily." On the other hand, there were such statements as, "Hiding and fleeing were a sort of adventure for us children," or "In a couple of days, I became a grown up person who always resists and fights for something. My motto is, One should never be panic-stricken!" In fact, this group of survivors is socially successful and well educated, at least half of them having earned university degrees.

EFFECT OF HOLOCAUST EXPERIENCES ON
RELIGIOUS ATTITUDES

As stated before, some of the interviewees declared that they have broken all ties with their religious beliefs, with God, and with ideals as a result of the Holocaust experiences, but they have remained Jews. A few became disillusioned with Jewishness because of some Jews' behavior in the camps— those who humiliated themselves, who stole things from one another, and who were brutal to other people, behaving barely better than the Germans. To my surprise, one musician said, "The *SS* men were cleaner and more handsome than the Jews."

The case of two half-Jewish sisters is worth describing. They were brought up as practicing Jews under the influence of Jewish grandparents, and survived by hiding in a convent where they converted to Catholicism. After the war, they declared themselves Jews, were members of the local Jewish community, married gentiles, and to this day feel torn between the two religions.

Indeed, a large proportion of the interviewees of both sexes intermarried with gentiles. It seems that Jews of mixed backgrounds show a tendency to marry partners who are also half-Jewish. A half-Jewish survivor, an editor, brought up far away from Jewish customs and culture, felt attracted to Jewishness only after having met a female writer (whom he later married) who was also a half-Jewish survivor. The woman's sister, a survivor as well, did not conceal her Jewish origin, but was never attracted to Jewish life and married a gentile.

POSSIBILITY OF A NEW HOLOCAUST

The interviewees continue to fear of the possibility of new ordeals as a consequence of their Jewish identity, though they worry less for themselves than for their children. A majority considers the state of Israel the best guarantee against such a possibility; others have confidence in their Christian friends, and some consider mixed marriages as an "antidote" against renewed antisemitism. Still others postulate two diametrically opposed solutions to the event of an outbreak of virulent antisemitism: emigration to Israel and total assimilation—though they do not consider the latter solution as a completely feasible one because of a perceived equivalence between anti-Israeli and anti-Jewish attitudes. Therefore, some Yugoslavian survivors do not exclude the possibility of a new Holocaust in their country.

THE SECOND GENERATION

Except for one family, the survivor population here gave no evidence of special problems in their offspring and found no Holocaust-related problems in their attitudes toward their own children. In the one exception, the mother blames the Holocaust for the deformity of her son's spine and for his kidney disease; she also indicated that her daughter should visit a psychiatrist. She stated, "The children are nervous." Several mothers said they were deliberately indulgent toward their children so as to compensate for the harshness they had had to endure.

Owing to the good organization of the Federation of Jewish Communities and the local communities, significant numbers of youngsters became active participants in the Jewish "youth-life." Their activities include seminars, gatherings, and summer holiday excursions. In the case of children of mixed marriages, their choice of affiliation depended greatly on parental influences.

Among the children of survivors, Jewish identity did not include an interest in survivor stories, and some, especially the children of mixed marriages, did not feel themselves as Jews at all. However, all are aware of being considered Jews by their countrymen "especially if something ugly happens." In my opinion, actual political events have influenced the ambivalent inner attitudes of many of the Jews and half-Jews who have remained disaffected until now (January 1993) because the sudden rise of interest in Jewishness does not seem to indicate a genuine interest in Jewish life, but rather a strategy to escape the civil war here by emigrating to Israel, and from there perhaps even further away.

FORGET AND FORGIVE

All the survivors, without exception, excluded the possibility of ever forgetting the Holocaust and its impact on their lives, and refused to forgive its perpetrators. Only a few of them considered forgiving the younger postwar generations of the German nation.

MOTIVATION, RESISTANCE, AND IMPACT

Approximately one-fifth of those invited refused to be interviewed out of fear of stirring up old, painful memories. Many felt that after more than forty years it is too late to arouse old memories and that no one is interested any longer in the past and present problems of the survivors. The husband of an interviewee tersely stated this view by citing the old Latin proverb: *"tarde venientibus ossa"* (for the late comers [to a banquet] only bones are left)!

Those who agreed to be interviewed expressed opinions about the interview's immediate impact, ranging from "a friendly chat," "a friendly cooperation, but also remembering unpleasant moments" to "Until now I have had nobody to speak to about this matter; I am very grateful, although it was painful. My husband (a gentile) does not allow me to speak about the camp, and my son is not interested in it." After my lengthy persuasion, a physician consented to speak as a friend and a colleague. "It was very painful," he said afterward, "but I feel an obligation towards this study. I suppress and dump a lot."

Almost all of the interviewed survivors emphasized that they were greatly motivated to participate in this study by the belief that what had happened to them should be known all over the world, so that such events will never happen again.

NOTES

1. Dr. Judith S. Kestenberg, founder with her husband, Milton Kestenberg (deceased), of the International Study of Organized Persecution of Children.

2. Since that time, the International Study of Organized Persecution of Children has affiliated with the psychology department at the Tel-Aviv University, where tapes are now available for academic research projects.

3. Editor's note [CK]: The editors do not concur completely with this global statement. While it is true that neither psychodynamic nor any other interview material can be reduced to "exact statistical" results, it is possible to organize, categorize, code, and quantify the content. At this writing, the Child Development Research group is actively engaged in the very process of coding hundreds of interviews with child survivors. The exploration of differences between quantitative and qualitative research began more than fifty years ago, resulting in a large number of articles, monographs, and books, addressing the issues of reliability, validity and measurement. See C. A. Landis, "A Statistical Evaluation of Psychotherapeutic Methods," in *Concepts and Problems of Psychotherapy*, ed. Leland F. Hinsie (New York: Columbia University Press, 1937); Lester Luborsky and Helen Sargent, "Sample Use of Method," *Bulletin of the Menninger Clinic* 20, no. 5 (1956): 263–76; Ann W. Shyne, ed., *Use of Judgments as Data in Social Research* (New York: National Association of Social Workers Conference, Research Section, 1959); Group for the Advancement of Psychiatry, "The Measurement of Change," *Psychiatric Research and Assessment of Change* 6, no. 63 (1966): 399–452; Helen Sargent, Leonard Horwitz, Robert Wallerstein, and Ann Appelbaum, "Prediction in Psychotherapy Research: A Method for the Transformation of Clinical Judgments into Testable Hypotheses," *Psychological Issues* 6, no. 1 (1968).

4. Editor's note [CK]: Never say never! Certainly not all personal shortcomings and failures are a consequence of Holocaust experiences. Yet, we know the long-lasting effects of trauma. Individual temperament, age and level of development, and the intensity of the traumatic experience interact and may well contribute to a failure of an individual's achievement of potentials. We wonder, too, whether the meaning

of the declaration "[shortcomings] are a private affair" is actually "a personal affair." In that case, we would have to agree; but "private" in the sense of secret? Why? Especially a psychiatrist must know that the better way of dealing with deficiencies is to try to correct them with the help of others, that is, the very opposite of keeping them private.

12

German-Jewish Identity

Charlotte Kahn

If anyone asked me where I belonged, my answer would be:
a Jewish mother brought me into this world,
Germany has nourished me,
Europe has educated me,
my home is this earth,
and the world my fatherland.[1]

A JEWISH GIRL IN NAZI GERMANY

On the platform at the railroad station one summer day in 1936, an eight-year-old girl and her father were waiting for the train to take them to the seashore in Holland. The girl, blue-eyed with long blonde braids, carried a knapsack. Her mother had nestled a baby doll inside, with its head and arms hanging out—much as mothers carry their real babies nowadays, but a spectacle in an era of baby buggies and doll carriages. A reporter took a photograph that appeared together with a four-stanza poem some weeks later in a Nazi newspaper, the *General Anzeiger*. The poem concluded with praise for the girl who will one day become a mother.[2] A German mother—presumably to bear children for the Führer.[3]

The irony is that the girl was a Jewish girl—indistinguishable in appearance from the non-Jewish Germans in her cohort.[4] Her trip to Holland was necessitated by the Nürnberg laws, which restricted German hotels to "Aryans." Jews were not allowed.

Two years later, that same Jewish girl proudly sported the Lyceum (girls' public, academic high school) school cap with hat band colors denoting her class. She was proud to have passed the entrance exam, proud to have been included, yet somewhat uncomprehending about why her classmates excluded her from games at recess. Had she offended anyone? She realized it had to do with her being Jewish and thought that on the Christians' part there was some misunderstanding about Jews. Wasn't she just like the other German girls, except that, instead of going to church on Sundays, she went to synagogue on Saturdays? She was conflicted, perhaps a little ashamed, about some family acquaintances' Jewish appearance, which reminded her of the caricatures in newspapers such as the *Stürmer*, but she never doubted the essence of being a Jew: Jewish ethics, rituals, or history. She was angry about being denigrated for reasons not at all logical to her. Only later, as an immigrant in England and the United States, did she feel truly second class: unprotected and fearful about being "stateless" (Nazi Germany having revoked the citizenship of Jewish emigrants); expecting discrimination because she was Jewish; cautious about speaking the "enemy's" language (i.e., German); and self-conscious about her accent, which betrayed her when speaking English.

I was that girl. Although I had been aware of aggressive antisemitism, it was only after experiencing the events of *Kristallnacht*—the burning synagogue, my uncle's arrest, my father's flight, the ravaging of our home and our escape across the garden wall into hiding in non-Jewish homes—that I realized that, as a group, Jews were going to be cast out of German society and that their Jewishness would take on primary importance. Our hyphenated identity was about to be ruptured.

Yes, I was a German Jew—as much German as Jew. During childhood, my identification with both parts of the hyphenated German-Jewish culture was equally strong: German and Jewish friends, German and Jewish caregivers, German high school preceded by Jewish elementary school. Through internalization of the patterns of my family's daily life, my sense of being German and being Jewish had become seamlessly fused. (It is not too different in the United States, where I am now an American-Jew.)

German and Jewish sensory experiences blended. The pastel colors of the north-European summer sky and the drab, gray winters; the shapes of the Gothic churches and of the Bauhaus features of my parents' home; and the smell of sausages were part of my life. But so were Chanukah lights; the interior of the synagogue with the white railing of the women's balcony (which, as a child, I was privileged to see both from below, sitting next to my father, as well as from above, when visiting the women); the smell of my grandfather's *havdalah* spices and candle, and the taste of *Berches*, the German-Jewish variation of *challah*. These sensory experiences represented loving connections that strongly influenced the "unconscious organizing structures of [my] interaction[s]."[5] I took my status for granted: German-Jewish, German albeit Jewish as well.

As a child in the 1930s, I had not been aware that German Jews— 600,000 of them, constituting .75 percent of a total German population of 80 million—were cognizant of their dual identification. A German-Jewish identity is characterized by a unique constellation of values and sociopsychological conditions. It grew out of the particular association between the Jewish minority and the German-speaking majority population. This association is characterized paradoxically by a cultural and commercial mutuality coupled variously with religious, political, national, and racial antisemitism.

GERMAN-JEWISH SYMBIOSIS

The establishment of a multiple identity, the hyphenated German-Jewish identity, can be accounted for partially by adducing the concept of symbiosis.[6] According to psychoanalytic principles, a symbiotic relationship is one of reciprocal need satisfaction. In contrast, separation from the enveloping symbiosis is a prerequisite for the establishment of an individual structure and a sense of identity.[7] The libidinal drive serves to bind objects, first symbiotically out of need and later in love. The aggressive drive serves the process of separation and differentiation. Aggression is used in the service of delineating a person, and later it becomes a protection against dissolution in a merger.

On a group level, parallel characteristics of symbiosis and separation in individual development can be observed in Jewish fusion with Germans, on the one hand, and their separate existence on the other. Cultural and economic need, together with some mutual admiration, were the underpinnings of a period of German-Jewish symbiosis. Antisemitism, driven by aggression, imposed separation on Jews and fostered the group's individuation toward a continuing, distinctly separate identity. Thus, at various times, Jews either chose to connect with or disassociate from the German culture, while Germans variously accepted or rejected them. Despite the conflict created by this paradox of closeness and distance, a significant number of famous people and, of course, many ordinary people, like myself, have identified themselves as German Jews. Giving up one or the other aspect of this set of identifications was equivalent to an amputation. The sensations in the stump of the amputated part remain.

German-Jewish identity has had a long history and continues even into the present—as my American-born children remind me from time to time, when they manifest typically German-Jewish tastes, attitudes, values, and an interest in mastering the German language. The long history of Jews in Germany began with their arrival in the German territories as physicians and traders, accompanying the Roman armies.[8] They lived side by side with the local population, experiencing not only oppression and persecution, but also tranquility and prosperity. Unlike France, England, and Spain after the expulsions, the German lands have never been totally devoid of Jews. In a not-yet unified Germany (prior to 1878), Jews who were expelled from one principality, duchy, or town moved to another.

During the late Middle Ages, Jews were forced into ghettos where they lived in quasi-autonomous Jewish communities *alongside*[9] the other members of the society. This physical separation and the heightened, aggressive, religious antisemitism that had been whipped up by the fervor of the Crusades, also separated Jews from Christian Germans psychologically. It strengthened Jewish identification with the Jewish culture that transcended the German boundaries. The late Middle Ages marked a period of separation-differentiation.

Centuries later, Jews interacted with the majority population, not only by virtue of having been invited by this king or that nobleman to carry out various financial tasks on their behalf. "Privileged" Jews, that is, those protected by nobles and kings, occupied a status comparable to non-Jewish freemen. The exception to this was their exemption from military service, insofar as that was predicated on land ownership, which had been proscribed for Jews.

ENLIGHTENMENT

The eighteenth-century European cultural development known as the Enlightenment was a crucial factor in the formation of the German-Jewish identity.

The Enlightenment affected many Jews of the time. They shed their cultural insularity sufficiently to include western European ideas in their tradition of learning. Despite considerable opposition among some Germans to the general philosophical and political changes in the direction of individual freedom, there prevailed the recognition that the subjugation of Jews was contradictory to the Enlightenment ideals of freedom, reason, and human dignity. As a result, the Enlightenment became a milestone in the bonding of the Jewish and the German cultures. Anticipating a seemingly "lasting fusion" that in the end was not realized, Jews began to live *with* the Germans.[10] In the cultured world of that time, Germans looked upon Jews as the spiritual and moral carriers of tradition.[11] In turn, Jews looked to the German culture as an avenue into the modern world. Some upper middle-class intellectual Germans and Jews became bound to each other in a cultural mutuality.

The German and Jewish cultural cross fertilization of the Enlightenment was exemplified by the intellectual and personal friendship, which commenced in 1756 between Gotthold Ephraim Lessing, the writer, and Moses Mendelssohn, the theologian. Lessing, the Christian, extolled a religion of reason, a Christianity purged of belief in biblical miracles and the supernatural character of Jesus. Mendelssohn, the Jew, demanded the elimination of mystical and superstitious ceremonies from the practice of Judaism. In 1755, embodying the Enlightenment ideal of the virtuous man, one committed to religious-metaphysical truth and ethical living, Moses Mendelssohn began to publish the journal *Preacher of Morals*.[12] Its counterpart was the Christian

journal *The Weekly Moral Writings*.[13] [14] Mendelssohn proclaimed the necessity for assimilation, exhorting Jews to relinquish ghetto habits and to
adapt to their greater surroundings. He expected that an increasingly reasonable and humanistic world would then treat Jews as equals.

The next milestone after the Enlightenment was the emancipation of the
German Jews, strongly influenced by the principles of the French Revolution. Emancipation was linked with the expectation of assimilation. This
view was expressed by Count Clermont-Tonnere, who earnestly suggested
that: "One must refuse the Jews everything as a nation and grant them
everything as individuals," implying that assimilation could—and in many
cases did—lead to baptism, or at least to an indifference toward Judaism.[15]
The Emancipation was, indeed, decisive in changing the Jews' sociological
status, as the emphasis shifted from the Jewish community to Jews as individuals. The Industrial Revolution and the demise of the guilds further fostered the German-Jewish economic symbiosis.

Beginning approximately in the mid–eighteenth century the "cooperation
of the Jews became a necessity in the new development of the German
economy."[16] In the free economy, Jews "filled certain gaps."[17]

Having been barred from tilling the soil and from the craft guilds, and
confined to petty trade, Jews had developed a combination of toughness
and flexibility in their personalities; in addition, they were industrious, frugal, and not prone to drink. Thus, they were prepared for the competitive,
mercantile life. By financing factories and starting enterprises in fields that
other businessmen were reluctant to enter, Jewish bankers and traders
forged an economic mutuality with the rising German bourgeoisie. Jews
became an integral part of a growing urban middle class.

Brilliant Jewish women of that era provided meeting places in their "sa-
lons," where Jewish and gentile intellectuals and aristocrats as well as young
radicals mingled. Among these women, Rahel Levin was probably the most
renowned. Born in 1771, she married Karl August Varnhagen von Ense, a
Prussian diplomat and author. He characterized her as "the third luminary
of Judaism, equalled in radiance by Jesus and Spinoza only." Rahel Levin-
Varnhagen was called "the first great modern woman in German cultural
life." And the poet Heinrich Heine believed her to be "the most gifted
woman of the universe."

Both Rahel Levin-Varnhagen and Heinrich Heine chose to be baptized.
Rahel's Jewishness embarrassed her; she idealized the German culture and
felt sullied by "the ignobility of her birth that placed an insuperable obstacle
in the way of her complete amalgamation with the aesthetic Germans."
Rahel tried to extricate herself from the "ignobility" of her Jewishness when,
in 1814, at age forty-four, she converted to Protestantism as a prerequisite
to her marriage.

As she familiarized herself with her newly adopted religion, Levin-
Varnhagen began to appreciate her Jewish roots, viewing Jesus as a brother,

a model of humility and love. Though she idealized and identified with the German culture, she could not shed her past. And because she continued to identify with the people of her birth, the anti-Jewish riots of 1819 in the provinces caused her even greater grief than her "ignoble birth." It seems that, in the end, she achieved the hyphenated German-Jewish identity, for she often intervened quietly on behalf of Jews and attempted to "wean" her non-Jewish friends from their "ingrained contempt" of Jews. In 1825, "she referred to herself as a 'refugee from Egypt and Palestine, who had found help and affection in Germany.'" That which had for so long " 'seemed my greatest disgrace . . . namely to have been born a Jewess, I would not now dispense with at any price.'" For his part, her husband August Varnhagen, deeply conscious of both Jewish cultural vitality and suffering, believed Jews truly to be God's chosen people.[18]

Heinrich Heine struggled with similar issues. His character was very nearly an amalgam of Jewish heredity and German environment. Heine superimposed the influence of Germany's philosophical currents upon his Jewish foundation. However, in a sense he was "the Jew awakened from his medieval dreams who, in his mad haste to adjust himself to the modern world, overstepped himself."[19] Heine's multiple identifications initially failed to coalesce into a hyphenated German-Jewish identity. Yearning for acceptance and success, he outwardly rejected Judaism and received a Christian baptism, not as a rite of conversion, but as representing "a ticket of admission to European culture." He resented the seemingly unavoidable necessity to submit to baptism, and considered it a stain on his honor. He attached no symbolic significance to baptism and expected to dedicate himself "all the more to the struggle for the rights of my racial comrades." When, after much doubt, he finally yielded for financial reasons, he did not cease to castigate himself and went so far as to attend a synagogue service in Hamburg to hear a sermon preached against Jews who abandon their faith for the hope of a job. Heine believed that "Jews must under all circumstances be preserved as an antidote to Christianity, which brings so much suffering to the mankind."[20]

Heine found a "spiritual affinity" with "ancient roots" between Jews and Germans. According to him, both had been "inexorable foes of the Romans . . . and the Bible, the great family chronicle of the Jews, served the entire Germanic world as an educational text." He referred to Germany as the "occidental Palestine" and to Palestine as the "oriental Germany." Noting differences between Jews and Germans, he recognized that, at the time, the German territories had not yet been forged into a fatherland, so that "Germans knew only loyalty to the leader or chieftain, migrating at his behest . . . while the Jews had . . . advanced beyond this stage and acknowledged loyalty solely to the moral code, the abstract principle of justice, universal law as embodied in the Torah."[21] Heine continued to the last to grapple with inner conflicts about his own multiple identities.[22]

Heine attributed German antisemitism to the fact that, by having "excluded Jews from agriculture and handicrafts," and compelling them to engage in trade and finance, "governments legally condemned Jews to be rich, hated, and ultimately murdered for plunder." In contrast, the German common people, farmers and artisans, whose choice of trade and profession had not been restricted, yearned for "the means of enjoying the present . . . [despite] the Christian insistence upon . . . renunciation of earthly goods."[23] With this, Heine approaches the point of view that the German-Jewish symbiosis ruptured at the point when the German *petit bourgeoisie* either no longer had a need for, or failed to keep pace with, the successful Jews.[24]

JEWS IN GERMANY AFTER EMANCIPATION

After the emancipation (beginning in 1808 at the behest of Napoleon Bonaparte, who had conquered the German territories), Jews gained admittance to German educational institutions and benefited greatly from their contacts with the German culture. At the same time, they contributed to it in a very large measure: Jews became "German *Gymnasiasten* [academic high school students] and German [university] students . . . *primum optimum* [of the first rank] . . . [and] respected colleagues in lawyers' chambers."[25]

Another measure of the continued symbiosis of the Jewish and German cultures is the extent to which Jews, prepared by their heritage of learning and their formerly restricted occupational opportunities, participated in the professional and scientific life in Germany. Konrad Jarausch notes that by 1932 there were 796 Jewish judges in Germany (except in Bavaria) and a Jewish Minister of Justice, Eugen Schiffer.[26] Law firms were often mixed, Jewish and gentile.[27] In 1933, when Jews constituted .75 percent of the Reich's population, 10 percent of all physicians were Jewish, while in Berlin 40 percent of the physicians were Jews.[28] [29] During the Weimar Republic, the Jewish industrialist and writer Walther Rathenau was appointed Minister of Interior and Minister of Reconstruction, with responsibility for aspects of the reparation policy (imposed on the Germans after World War I by the Treaty of Versailles). He had earlier been instrumental in founding the middle-class Democratic Party.[30]

By 1933, of the twenty Jewish Nobel Prize winners in the world,[31] fifteen had come from German-speaking territories; that is, when Hitler ascended to power, members of the small group of German Jews had won 9 percent of the total number of Nobel Prizes (170) granted worldwide.[32]

In the fields of the arts and humanities, Jews were indebted to "German circles which, since the Enlightenment, had opened for the Jews the gates to modern life."[33] Appreciative of the energy and enthusiasm that Jews invested in promoting new ideas, the gentile author, Annette Kolb, wrote in

1934, "We are a little flock of Christians in Germany today who remain aware of their debt of gratitude to Jewry."[34]

ANTISEMITISM

An ever-present antisemitism also underwent changes in concordance with historical and economic events: During the Middle Ages, a Jew could reduce the aggression of religious antisemitism and the distance between himself and the gentile community by baptism. Later, religious hatred changed to something resembling political discrimination based partially on economic envy. Only with the rise of Romanticism and nationalism did antisemitism become ethnic, that is, *völkisch*. This was the basis for the Nazi racist theories—from which there was no escape.

Confronting the inexorable antisemitism, German Jews organized themselves as a separate group to protect their specific communal rights and interests. As early as 1819 a group of seven young men had formed the "society for the improvement of the Jewish condition in the German states." These intellectuals had previously assembled to revamp their thinking about Judaism. They needed to synchronize their Jewish identity with their life and identity as modern Germans. They called their approach the Science of Judaism.[35] They named their think-tank the "Union of Jews for Culture and Science in 1821."[36] Heinrich Heine joined this group in 1822.

The Central Association of German Citizens of Jewish Faith, the "CV," came into existence in 1893.[37] The purpose of the CV was to "come together to work for . . . civil and social equality, as well as for the cultivation of . . . German-mindedness."[38] In the very year it was organized, the CV also "established a legal defence commission[39] . . . to act through the courts against antisemitic actions and publications."[40] The CV organization attempted to protect its Jewish membership. Yet, aggression in the form of antisemitism continued to sharpen the boundaries between Jews and other Germans, thus reaffirming the separate and distinctly Jewish identity.

As a group, Jews did not amalgamate with and disappear within the larger Christian society. Continuing antisemitism was one factor preventing total assimilation. Strong family loyalties, identification with Jewish cultural and ethical values, and, for some, religious conviction were other reasons. Although Jews were in close association with Germans, imposed and chosen separation coalesced to assure a continuing Jewish identity.

GERMAN-JEWISH IDENTITY

German Jews had forged a synthesis out of their identities. The bonding of Jewish tradition and German philosophy, and its subsequent internalization, constituted an important part of the core of the hyphenated German-Jewish identity. As Jews they had lived through the period of economic and cultural symbiosis without losing themselves in a total merger. They acculturated to their surroundings, and they committed themselves politically to the country of their birth. In this way, as a group, Jews accomplished their developmental tasks of separation-individuation and the establishment of a meaningful, if time-limited, relationship with the Germans. Having endowed both their self- and object-representations with value, they formed a multiple identity that seemed viable at the time. Thus, when he learned of the Russian pogroms of 1905, Georg Tietz, a wealthy department store owner, reflected on his identity as a Jew. Concluding that he was a Jew in the ethical sense and a German politically and culturally, he decided to "give unto the Kaiser what is due to the Kaiser and to God what is due to God." Then he prayed that he would never have to confront the question, whether he was Jew or German.[41]

For Tietz's descendants, the question was posed and answered by German antisemitism. The complete dissolution of the German-Jewish symbiosis was effected by the course that antisemitic virulence took in twentieth-century Germany. A confluence of factors seems to have spurred this intense, organized antisemitism: Germans needed a tribal romanticism to establish a sense of unity among the disparate groups within the German-speaking territories when they belatedly began to function as a nation in the context of the Kaiser Reich and subsequently in the Third Reich.[42] The romantically tinged *völkisch* (ethnic) emphasis on tribalism reinforced the existing religious antisemitism, which, for two millenia, had taught Christian children that Jews were Christ-killers. Their sense of tribal unity made it easy for the Germans to exclude the Jews. Furthermore, the frequently-cited German authoritarian personality, added to the German public's political inexperience (a consequence of rule by the aristocracy and the lack of a meaningful popular vote), left the population vulnerable to the *völkisch* antisemitism of the Weimar period. Also, at that time of the German people's humiliation and suffering, immediately after World War I, and during the subsequent periods of economic inflation and depression, the envious *petit bourgeoisie* needed—and found—a convenient scapegoat in that more successful, easily distinguishable group amongst them, the Jews. Thus was the stage set for National Socialism and the Holocaust.

The Nazis destroyed a blossoming culture in Germany, spawned by a fusion of the best of the German and the Jewish spirits. They destroyed this singular culture developed over the course of the centuries of Jewish life in Germany.[43] "The Jews were the good conscience of the [German] nation. Through their presence, the Jews became a moral factor—representatives of a universal human ethic, of the grand idea of '*Humanité*' and all that is connected with it."[44]

As traumatic and disruptive as deportation and emigration were, most surviving German Jews in exile clung to their civilized ways. For example, the poet Alfred Mombert, son of a physician and himself a nonpracticing lawyer, was deported in 1940 to a concentration camp in Gurs, France. There he wrote

The Darkness

Barracks, winter, darkness
. . . Phantoms of lunacy:
would feud with me!
fight against me!
Would destroy me: the symbol!
Justice will come—the final judgment.
Already it stares at you!!—
I will not stop the great last judgment!!—
Chaos-filth—the morass of death
oozed from the suppurating dragon—
rolls along my lily pond—
before God's glowing fortress
you exult around my Garden of Hesperides—
—The scourge on you—muck on you—then fire!
Night-ash on the lips—
bitter—bitter—
But triumph in spirit . . .
—Yet like a wreath around my body
now wraps in barrack-darkness
Satan: chain-demon— . . .
Night-ash on the lips—
bitter—bitter—
But triumph in spirit.[45]

Though often stunted by terror and torture, denigration and dislocation, the spirit triumphed. Sensual and emotional experiences, rooted in the German landscape and lifestyle, and seasoned with the Jewish traditions, were often relived, recounted, even recreated. The individual identification with the German-Jewish culture—its philosophy, art, and science—was fortified, and to this day, the group identity is affirmed when German Jews get together. They read and discuss, and often use expressions special to them. They pun and joke in ways that are incomprehensible to others, and savor foods and smells that seem not particularly delicious to others. They refer to places and events that are meaningful to them alone: not to Americans, not to German gentiles, not even to other Jews.

The German-Jewish culture molded me. Then, exiled from Germany into strange environments, I felt betrayed, disoriented, and denigrated. Yet, the values of the German-Jewish culture sustained and guided me. Focusing on the achievements of my cultural ancestors helped to heal my wounded pride and pointed to my future responsibility. Integrated with my American-Jewish identity, the German-Jewish identity lives on in me. Fainter traces continue to color my children's lives. For my grandchildren, German-Jewish culture will have receded into the history books.

NOTES

1. Ernst Toller, "Eine Jugend in Deutschland" (1933) quoted in Solomon Liptzin, *Germany's Stepchildren* (1944; Cleveland and New York: The World Publishing Co., 1961), 201. Toller (1896–1939) was a writer and pacifist.
    2.

> Ohne Puppe keinen Schritt!
> Ob sie nun Lottchen heißt, ob Gretchen,
> Sie ist ein ganz patentes Mädchen,
> Denn sie hat Herz und hat Gemüt,
> Geht ohne Püppchen keinen Schritt.
>
> Ihr Puppenkindchen hat es gut,
> Selbst wenn sie eine Reise tut,
> Zum Wochenende beispielsweise,
> Dann nimmt Sie es mit auf die Reise.
> Und anstatt in den Rucksack nun,
> Was Leckeres hineinzutun,
> So Kuchen, Obst, auch Brot und Butter,
> Wie man so sagt, das Reisefutter,
> Guckt aus dem Rucksack anstatt Schmaus,
> Das gut gepflegte Püppchen 'raus.
>
> Ja, ja, hier zeigt sich zart und still,
> Was einst 'ne Mutter werden will!

Huba, *General Anzeiger*, August 1936.
    3. "Nazi women extolled motherhood . . . [and] Nazi doctrine enforced selective breeding." Women were to carry out "Hitler's plan for a genetically superior . . . generation." This included the "unwed mothers who bore children for the Führer"; they earned Himmler's special praise. Claudia Koonz, *Mothers in the Fatherland* (New York: St. Martin's Press, 1987), 285, 306, 398.
    4. In 1938 a non-Jewish, anti-Nazi photographer submitted the picture of the baby daughter of Jakob and Pauline Levinsons, a Latvian-Jewish couple living in Berlin. The picture won first prize and appeared in the newspaper as well as on greeting cards. (Personal communication.) See also Hessy Levinsons-Taft, "Perfect Aryan," in *Muted Voices, Jewish Survivors of Latvia Remember*, ed. Gertrude Schneider (New York: Philosophical Library, 1987), 112–18.
    5. Lawrence Selnick and Esther Buchholz, "The Concept of Mental Representations in Light of Recent Infant Research," *Psychoanalytic Psychology* 7 (1990): 29–58, quote cited on 29.
    6. Adolf Leschnitzer, *The Magic Background of Modern Antisemitism* (New York: International Universities Press, 1956).
    7. Margaret Mahler, "Separation and Individuation," in *The Psychoanalytic Study of the Child*, 53 vols. (New York: International Universities Press, 1963).

8. Konrad Schilling, ed., *Monumenta Judaica: 2000 Jahre Geschichte und Kultur der Juden am Rhein* (2000 years history and culture of the Jews at the Rhein) (Stadt Köln, Germany: Bechem Drucker, 1963).

9. Leschnitzer, *Magic Background*, 26.

10. Ibid.

11. *"Kulturträger."*

12. *Kohelet Musar.*

13. *"Moralische Wochenschriften."*

14. "When pronounced in German, *'Juden und Aufklärung'* (Jews and Enlightenment) has a special resonance"; they are the opening words of a 1992 article by David Sorkin in the *Leo Baeck Institute Yearbook*. David Sorkin, "Jews, the Enlightenment and Religious Toleration—Some Reflections," in *Leo Baeck Institute Yearbook XXXVII*, ed. Arnold Paucker (London: Secker & Warburg, 1992), 3–16.

15. Wolfgang Benz, "The Legend of German-Jewish Symbiosis," in *Leo Baeck Institute Yearbook XXXVII*, ed. Arnold Paucker (London: Secker & Warburg, 1992), 95.

16. Leschnitzer, *Magic Background*, 16–17, 27.

17. Ibid., 7.

18. Liptzin, *Germany's Stepchildren*, 7–16

19. Ibid., 68.

20. Ibid., 68–71.

21. Ibid., 76ff.

22. Heine's predictions of conflict among nations and socioeconomic classes, and his anticipation of struggles among religious groups turned out to be amazingly accurate. Liptzin, *Germany's Stepchildren*, 80. Although this is not the place to discuss this topic, one may wonder about how much of Heinrich Heine found its way into Freud's "Group Psychology and the Analysis of the Ego" (1921), in *The Standard Edition of the Complete Psychological Works of Sigmund Freud* (London: The Hogarth Press, 1955), 18:69–144.

23. Liptzin, *Germany's Stepchildren*.

24. Leschnitzer, *Magic Background*, 91ff.

25. Benz allows that 100,000 German Jews, bonded to the fatherland, served in the First World War—a high proportion of the Jewish population of 550,000 at the time. Twelve thousand of them were killed in battle. Benz, "Legend of German-Jewish Symbiosis."

26. Konrad Jarausch, "Jewish Lawyers in Germany, 1848–1938—The Disintegration of a Profession," in *Leo Baeck Institute Yearbook XXXVI*, ed. Arnold Paucker (London: Secker & Warburg, 1991), 171–90.

27. 48.3 percent of Berlin lawyers were Jewish; in Frankfurt, 45.3 percent. 9.4 percent of the general university enrollment in 1894/1895 was Jewish, although they then constituted less than 1 percent (.91 percent) of the population. This proportion had declined by 1932, as a result of fewer Jewish births.

28. Geoffrey Cocks, "Partners and Pariahs—Jews and Medicine in Modern German Society," in *Leo Baeck Institute Yearbook XXXVI*, ed. Arnold Paucker (London: Secker & Warburg, 1991), 191–205.

29. Although after the Nürnberg Laws of 1935 "Aryans" were not permitted to consult Jewish physicians, they were held in high regard, as I know from a sad personal experience. In 1935 the newly introduced diphtheria vaccine maintained its

efficacy for a relatively short period of time. As a result, a Christian playmate, who lived in the house next door, contracted the disease; I did, too. When I returned from the hospital, I learned that the boy had died. His mother cried to mine, "If only we had had a good Jewish doctor!"

30. *Encyclopædia Britannica*, vol. 18 (1965), 990ff.

31. Fourteen Jewish and six with one Jewish parent

32. Leschnitzer, *Magic Background*, 217.

33. Ibid., 51.

34. Ibid.

35. *Wissenschaft des Judentums* and *Verein für Cultur und Wissenschaft der Juden* was the name of the organization.

36. Ismar Schorsch, "Breakthrough into the Past: The *Verein für Cultur und Wissenschaft der Juden*," in *Leo Baeck Institute Yearbook XXXIII*, ed. Arnold Paucker (London: Secker & Warburg, 1988), 3.

37. *Centralverein deutscher Staatsbürger Jüdischen Glaubens.*

38. *Deutsche Gesinnung.*

39. *Rechtsschutzkommission.*

40. Evyatar Friesel, "The *Centralverein* and the American Jewish Committee: A Comparative Study," in *Leo Baeck Institute Yearbook XXXVI*, ed. Arnold Paucker (London: Secker & Warburg, 1991), 102.

41. Werner Mosse, "Integration and Identity in Imperial Germany: Towards a Typology," in *Leo Baeck Institute Yearbook XXXVII*, ed. Arnold Paucker (London: Secker & Warburg, 1992), 83–93.

42. Ismar Schorsch, "Breakthrough into the Past: The *Verein für Cultur und Wissenschaft der Juden*," in *Leo Baeck Institute Yearbook XXXIII*, ed. Arnold Paucker (London: Secker & Warburg, 1988), 3.

43. Although an active Jewish community still exists in Germany now, almost all its members are World War II displaced persons and their descendants, or recent immigrants. My readings and observations indicate that these post–World War II Jews have brought with them other cultural variants, and remain rightfully wary of German antisemitism. The Jews now living there lack the protracted, uninterrupted experience of life in Germany.

44. *Die Juden waren das gute Gewissen der Nation. Durch ihre Präsanz waren die Juden ein moralischer Faktor—Vertreter einer universellen Menschheitsethik, der gro-ßen Idee der 'Humanite' und all dessen, was mit ihr verbunden ist. Johannes Rau. Zum Geleit* (Jews were the conscience of the nation. Through their very presence they became a moral factor—representative of a universal human ethic, the grand idea of a "humanity" and all that is connected with it) [transl. C.K.], in *Juden als Träger Bürgerlicher Kultur in Deutschland*, ed. Julius H. Schoeps (Bonn, Germany: Burg Verlag, 1989), 37.

45. *In der Finsternis*

Baracken, Winter, Finsternis
. . . Fantom aus Wahn-Geschichte:
wolltest wider mich streiten!
streitest wider mich!
Willst zerstören mich: das Sinn-Bild!
Gericht Kommt!—Ende-Gericht!

Schon starrt es dich an!!
Aufhalten werd' ich nicht das große, letzte Gericht!!—
Chaos-Kot—der Morast des Todes
entkrochen eitriger Drachen—
wältztest heran an meinen kastalischen Quell
vor der erglühten Götter-Burg
jauchzt du um meinen Garten der Hesperiden—
—die Geißel dir—dir Fraß—und dann Feuer!—
Nacht-Asche auf den Lippen—
bitter—bitter—
but Triumph im Geist
—Aber mir um den Leib als Kranz die Kette
schlang jetzt in Baracken-Finsternis
Satan: Ketten-Dämon— . . .
Nacht-Asche auf den Lippen—
bitter—bitter—
aber Triumph im Geist.

Alfred Mombert, *In der Finsternis* [emphasis and trans. Charlotte Kahn], in *Monumenta Judaica* (Köln, Germany: Konrad Schilling, 1963), 496.

13

Kindertransport: A Case Study

Judith S. Kestenberg

Ten thousand children were sent to England from Germany, Austria, Czechoslovakia and a few from other countries.[1] Some were three year olds and even younger. Some went alone, others with sisters or brothers. They were brought to the train by mothers and fathers who did not cry, but smiled instead. And off they went into the unknown. All were scared. Accompanying them were young men or women who took care of them and told them what to do at the border. They also saw to it that they played. Some girls, perhaps the majority, had dolls tucked under their arms, a reminder of home. What happened to them when they arrived in London?

Most of the children were placed with families, some Jewish and some not Jewish. The latter were raised as Protestants and most of them remained so. The younger ones forgot their mothers and became attached to their foster mothers. At first their mothers wrote to them, but when war broke out in September 1939, the writing stopped. Only a few were reunited with their families after the war. Most lost their parents and siblings. Perhaps the following case of a *Kindertransport* child will bring these children to life for the reader, place in context the difficulties they faced, and formulate the some as-yet-unanswered questions.

Gisa was seven years old when she came to England. She remembers the many children and the chaos on the train. She does not remember her mother, father, or her two older brothers. She had been told she was going to her sister in Scotland, but her sister never appeared. After a few days in London, she was "shipped" to a Scottish hospital that had been converted into a Jewish orphanage. There she remained with others, almost all older than herself, but sharing her fate. These children were hungry (as all of England was hungry), and it was cold because there was a fuel shortage. An active child, Gisa never froze, but other children suffered frostbite.

Remarkably, she neither remembered nor missed her mother and the two brothers she had left in Germany, and she does not remember seeing her sister—although the sister must have visited her, because she later told Gisa that she was a crying, disheveled child. Her memory is of toughness—she was not worried or depressed. How did this happen to a seven year old?

Before leaving for England she had been placed in a German orphanage, where she squabbled with her older brothers. It almost seems that she so much resented her family for "abandoning" her that she erased them from her conscious memory. What about her sister? All the way to Scotland Gisa had been looking forward to meeting her, but when she finally came, it was too late. Gisa no longer remembered her sister's visits. She remembered only that she did not want anybody to pity her because she was tough. She never cried in front of people, but she did cry in bed when no one would see or hear her. Did she put this stamp of pride and self-sufficiency on her early childhood as a symbol of her toughness, as if to say, not she, only others cried—the weak people? This idea runs through the entire, long interview.

Because she performed well in school, Gisa was allowed to continue her education while staying with Jewish foster families, who were paid to care for her. She complained that they made her wash dishes and wash the floor, and perform all functions of servitude. After a succession of foster homes, she landed in the house of a British couple with a baby. They let her do what she wanted. She remained in school until the last grade, when in restlessness she dropped out, and at age sixteen she went to Israel to live on a *kibbutz*. On the *kibbutz*, she had many boyfriends—to the despair of the bachelors. However, she became especially attached to a *madrich* (a leader) who was suffering the aftereffects of poliomyelitis and was confined to doing paperwork. He listened to her and became her substitute father. He even gave her money from his reparation payments when she finally decided to leave the *kibbutz*. Later, when he died, she cried.

Wanting to be tough like men, Gisa joined the Israeli army and was assigned to a noncommissioned officers' school where she trained the soldiers. At the end of her two-year military duty, instead of joining the officers' school, she left. Subsequently, she suffered depressed moods for three months. She did not know what to do next. Similar experiences have been reported by the child survivors who used the military as a temporary support. It provided a holding environment, replacing the homes these young people had lost. They felt as lost leaving the military as they did leaving their families.[2]

One of her friends was a veterinarian who helped her obtain a job elsewhere. These were glorious years. She rented her own apartment—a home, so very important to her. Soon she met her future husband, with whom she went to the United States. Even though he was wonderful and they laughed a lot together, she could not stand his rigidity and his bossiness. After a year she divorced him and then had several boyfriends, who lived separately from her. All her friends must have been older than she, because, with the exception of her husband, all died long before she grew old. Gisa believes she lacks the capacity for intimacy. She likes to be alone, to read and to write, though she does not get published. Now Gisa regrets not having worked and saved enough for her old age, and plans to commit suicide when she can no longer work.

Gisa traveled a lot, as if trains held an attraction for her. Using it as a symbol of separation, the train surrounded by children appears also in her nightmares. Repeatedly she put herself into a victim role, perhaps repeating earlier frightening experiences. For example, she remembers a man coming into the bathroom window of her home, while she was taking a bath during *Kristallnacht* (the Night of Broken Glass). Whether this actually happened is not important, for it may be a screen memory covering other dangerous situations from which she miraculously escaped.

She has asked a beloved uncle for information about her mother and father. She believes that she looks like her mother, whereas her sister looks more like their non-Jewish father. Gisa has always accepted her Jewishness, but has no children to pass on the legacy of Judaism. Her sister, on the other hand, married a Jew and has four children, but never talks to them about what happened to her. She forbade Gisa to speak to the children about the Holocaust. Gisa speculates that the sister is ashamed either of Gisa's having been a *Kindertransport* child or of their father's non-Jewish origins.

In contrast, Gisa speaks about her experiences, the more so since the convention of *Kindertransport* children two years prior to the interview. While she can now talk about it, she worries most (although, typically, she does not admit to it) about how tough she had to be, how alone she was, and that she did not stay with any of the people who wanted to marry her.

Gisa has not always been alone, having been *with* a man several times over. She admits to wanting to *be* a man, to be tough. Once, when the Canadians parachuted into Paris, she followed a group of children with parasols who jumped off a roof, and she broke her leg. She had three operations, and to this day seems to be accident prone. The first operation occurred during her childhood, making her particularly aware that she lacks a mother. To compensate, she prides herself on her capacity to have many, many friends. Can it be that the accidents and illnesses both recreate and cover up her longing for mother as well as for a family of her own?

What does this *Kindertransport* child tell us about herself? She longs for parents and seeks father substitutes in older men. She befriends other peoples' children rather than having her own. Beneath the veneer of toughness she seems to punish herself. For what? For having survived? For forgetting her mother in revenge for her mother's abandoning her? While some *Kindertransport* children openly confess that they felt abandoned by their mothers, Gisa seems to abandon herself. Did she become so isolated, so alone, and so tough because she lacked parents or to protect her vulnerability? Or does she feel abandoned by her parents, who kept the two brothers, but sent the two girls away? Over and over again she maneuvers to be abandoned. She divorced her husband. She left an alcoholic whom she had loved. The other men died. And the abandonment continues.

Is the train of her nightmares a symbol of abandonment? One could speak of her experience as "abandonment with many children." At the *Kindertransport* reunion she was once more surrounded by her old friends, who accepted rather than rejected her, and the subsequent formation of a *Kindertransport* association has done her a world of good. She feels very strongly that she was lucky not to have been placed with a family immediately upon arriving in England, because her first foster family did not treat her well. The institution treated all children very well, despite the pervasive hunger and cold. Unfortunately, one woman who seemed to have been especially warm and kind died. Throughout her life, Gisa's close friends died, either by accident or because she chose older mates.

Is Gisa repeating her trauma by becoming attached to people who are apt to die? Perhaps she is too tough to become attached to anyone, for she mourns no one except her substitute father. (She had no way of knowing her biological father who went into hiding when she was still a baby.)

Kindertransport children were often were mistreated by their caretakers, who as a group were not trained in parenting. Separating children from siblings as well as from parents often results in a later inability to form attachments and engage in intimate relationships.[3] This does not mean that no *Kindertransport* children were able to marry. Many of them did, especially if they were old enough at the time of the separation to remember their parents, which made it easier to form attachments.

NOTES

1. Dorit Bader Whiteman, *The Uprooted: A Hitler Legacy* (New York: Plenum Press, 1993).

2. Editor's note [CK]: Similar reactions are quite common among discharged soldiers who are not survivors. Even retirees from a career-military service often find themselves at loose ends, anxious, and are temporarily unable to discharge their civilian and family duties. It is as if the structure of the military had functioned in the place of an internalized executive ego.

3. Anna Freud and Sophie Dann, "An Experiment in Group Upbringing," in *The Psychoanalytic Study of the Child*, 53 vols. (New York: International Universities Press, 1951), 6: 127–68; E. Papanek and E. Linn, *Out of the Fire* (New York: William Morrow, 1975).

14

Sweden and the Holocaust

Hedi Fried

Displaced persons
We have no heart. . . .
Fate broke it
in pieces.
Born as strangers
in our own mother tongue,
transported as a race
to the land of Germans
. . . after the landslide, only shambles . . .
Married to a Pole
did you remain Jewish?
Married to a Swede
did you become Swedish?
Married to a German!
That you can never forget . . .
The iron curtain cuts through
your own family album.
What do you say to your children
Who are you?[1]

HISTORICAL FLASHBACK

Sweden, a neutral country during World War II, played an important role in the rescue and rehabilitation of some European Jews. Sweden's first contact with Jews can be traced back to the Viking trade with the Khazars on the Crimean. However, before the end of the eighteenth century, only converted Jews were allowed in Sweden. The Lutheran Swedes, who wanted to protect their faith, did not let Jews settle. One exception was Dr. Benedictus de Castro (Baruch Nehemias), who had been invited by Queen Christina in 1645. A few others, among them the Jewish creditors of Charles XII, who followed him from Turkey in 1715, received permission to stay for ten years. Still, in 1741, a decree forbade residence to "all Jews, Savoyards, equilibrists, comedians, and other jesters, whatever their name, Tatars and Gypsies who cause the community inconvenience and all kind of trouble through their ungodliness, soothsayings, lies, and theft." However, with the accession to the throne of the enlightened King Gustaf III, the situation slowly changed.

The first Jew to arrive under his reign in 1774 was Aaron Isaac, a seal-engraver from Mecklenburg, who received permission to practice his religion. When he explained that this could be done only in a congregation (*minyan*), ten more Jews were allowed to enter. Thus, a Jewish community was slowly formed on the west coast of Sweden. The king, a well-traveled man aware of the important role Jews played at the different royal courts in Europe, influenced the Parliament to grant them the right to settle in Stockholm, Göteborg, and Norrköping. The 1782 regulations, governing Jews who wished to enter the country, were modeled after those in other European countries, but were somewhat more liberal. Accordingly, while the Jews lived only in the above-mentioned three cities, they were allowed to conduct religious services, acquire real estate, and engage in trades not subject to the guilds. They were an autonomous community of foreigners to whom intermarriage with Swedes was proscribed. Not until 1838, when a royal decree abolished the autonomy of the Jews and named them "Mosaic communities, adherents of the Mosaic faiths," were the Jews incorporated into the Swedish state. This decree aroused strong opposition as some antisemitic feelings also prevailed and, therefore, it had to be modified. Nevertheless, it represents the beginning of the political emancipation of the Swedish Jews, and it remained in force until 1957.

In 1838, Jews in Sweden numbered only 900 souls. Slowly, all restrictions on occupations and intermarriage were lifted, and in 1870 Jews were granted the right to settle all over Sweden and even to hold political office, provided they join the Swedish state church. Thus emancipation and assimilation advanced, without any interference from the growing antisemitism manifested in other parts of Europe. As a result, religious life among Swedish Jews declined, and several Jewish musicians, painters, and literary critics emerged. The somnolent Jewish life was revived by immigrants from Eastern Europe who made their way to Sweden between 1860 and 1933.

In that period, the ordinary Swedish people were seldom antisemitic, as they knew very little about Jews. However, being so isolated, they knew very little about any foreigners, and apparently feared them. Thus, they have been very xenophobic for centuries. In 1927, following the ideas of racial purity prevailing at the time, one proposition of a new law regarding foreigners stated: "The value of the unusual homogeneity and purity of the population of our country can hardly be exaggerated." This resulted in

Jews being looked upon as foreigners, even though some of them had been Swedish citizens for more than a hundred years, and explains the Swedish animosity towards Jews as generally xenophobic rather than specifically antisemitic.

HOLOCAUST PERIOD

After Hitler's rise to power, the Jews tried to persuade the Swedish government to rescue their German brethren. However, as the economic situation in Sweden was very bad, there was no positive response. The fear of competition for jobs, and of arousing a so far almost nonexistent antisemitism, resulted in a refusal to grant entry permits, despite the imminent danger to the German Jews. Sweden and Switzerland asked Germany to have Jewish passports marked with the letter "J" to make it easier to reject Jewish applicants. Sybilla, the wife of the Swedish Prince Royal was of German origin, and thus the royal family, the high military dignitaries, and the upper classes had pro-German sympathies. Consequently, very few Jews were allowed to enter the country before the outbreak of the war.

Nevertheless, at the end of 1938 and during 1939, about 650 German-Jewish children aged two to sixteen arrived in Sweden with the so-called *Kindertransport* (children's transport). Although these children were the responsibility of the Jewish community who initiated this immigration, 150 converted children were taken care of by the Israel Mission. Some of them were adopted by Swedish families, Jewish and gentile; others stayed in camps especially organized for them. Some camps were modeled after Swedish children's camps, others aimed to prepare the children for immigration to Israel.

Strictly speaking, Sweden had no hidden children. Those who had been in hiding arrived in Sweden at different stages in their lives, most of them in adulthood. Many of the children who survived the concentration camps arrived from Bergen Belsen after the war. Some, like Isaac, had survived Auschwitz.

Isaac was born in 1930 and, having survived Auschwitz all alone, arrived in Sweden in 1945 at the age of fifteen. He was very weak, and after two months of convalescence did not weigh more than forty kilos (88 pounds). As he remembers, as soon as the allotted two months had passed, he was put into a factory to work. He remembers being very lonely and miserable, having no one to talk to or to help him, economically or psychically. Isaac never had an opportunity to study and continued to be a factory worker for many years. He feels he was mistreated when he arrived in Sweden in that he was not given any support or education.

In contrast, Jacob, who also survived Auschwitz, was born in 1936 and arrived in Sweden with his parents in 1948, at the age of twelve.[2] Jacob attended school, quickly learned Swedish, developed into a strong and capable young boy, and worked his way through a technical school, attaining the title of "technical engineer." He believes having his mother near him in the concentration camp gave him a sense of security despite the hardships, and his childhood experiences turned him into a fighter with a will to survive.[3] He mentioned that he succeeded despite having received no help from either the Swedish or Jewish communities.

During the war, when the Nazi atrocities became known and when the unemployment problem turned into a shortage of workers, public opinion began to improve. Still, the government was afraid to spoil its good relationship with Hitler. However, in 1942 the first Jewish refugees were allowed to cross the border during the invasion of Norway and half of the Norwegian-Jewish population was rescued. One year later, with the invasion of Denmark, public opinion changed completely, and a most efficient cooperation between Swedes and Danes resulted in the rescue of the entire Danish-Jewish population. During one night, all the 8,000 Danish Jews, plus the German refugees living in Denmark, were transported by fishermen in small fishing boats through the straits between Denmark and Sweden.

In 1944, at the request of Jewish authorities, a young Swedish diplomat, Raoul Wallenberg, was sent to Hungary to rescue Jews. By issuing Swedish *Schutzpässe* (protective passports), he was able to save a large number of Hungarian Jews. At about the same time, the Norwegian government in exile approached the Swedish government, asking them to rescue Norwegian citizens from the concentration camps. Count Folke Bernadotte was appointed to initiate action toward this end, and his endeavors resulted in Himmler's consent to release all Norwegian and Danish prisoners. In March 1944, the action later known under the name of "the white buses" started. Volunteers in ambulances marked with a large red cross started to transport the Scandinavians from Sachsenhausen, Dachau, and Mauthausen, while the U.S. Air Force subjected Germany to heavy bombing.

Early in 1945, when the war was nearing its end, the World Jewish Congress, under the leadership of Gilel Storch, chairman of the Swedish branch of the World Jewish Congress, also initiated a contact with Germany, through Himmler's favorite masseur, Felix Kersten. The aim was to save the remaining Jews in the concentration camps from a feared final execution. This resulted in a historical meeting between Himmler and the Swedish Jew, Norbert Masur. By the end of 1944, Himmler no longer believed in victory. Without informing Hitler, he entered into negotiations with Gilel Storch. Himmler's belief in the power of the Jews was so strong, and his fear of them so great, that he absolutely believed the head of the World Jewish Congress to be the most powerful man in Sweden. Thus, he invited him to a personal meeting, and on April 19, 1945, the unbelievable happened: While the Allies were continuously bombing Germany, a Jew landed under a safe conduct at the Berlin airport. However, owing to special circumstances, the person that crossed the border was not Gilel Storch, a refugee from the Baltic, but Norbert Masur. After some dramatic hours, the meeting with Himmler took place, resulting in Himmler's accepting all the demands of the Jew, without even asking for anything in return. Parcels of food and medicine were allowed to be sent into the camps, and the Swedish buses were allowed to rescue Norwegian Jews from Grini and Ravensbrück, and additional Jews from Theresienstadt. Himmler also promised that no more transports would take place and no camps would be liquidated. The next day, the white buses arrived at Ravensbrück to rescue the Norwegian Jews. There they were told to take whomever they wanted, and thus 10,000 non-Norwegian Jewish women were included in this transport. This was in March 1945. One month later, the advancing English troops stumbled upon the concentration camp of Bergen-Belsen, which then turned out to be the first camp to be liberated on April 15, 1945.

After the end of the war, May 7, 1945, Sweden continued its humanitarian work and decided to bring in the sick from Bergen-Belsen for a two-month convalescence. The plan was to give them medical assistance and afterward help them travel back to their countries of origin. Several thousand of these very sick people had been transported to Sweden on stretchers and placed in hospitals and sanatoria. Quite a number died of tuberculosis (TB) and other diseases, but many recovered. Those who stayed were slowly absorbed by the nation.

The sick were allowed to be accompanied by their families, who were quarantined all over the country in provisional camps, empty schools, museums, and so forth. The Jewish community tried to organize visits to hospitals and camps, but could hardly meet the needs of the new arrivals. Community members traveled around Sweden, handing out small items such as combs, pens, and lipsticks—items symbolizing that these people were once again looked upon as human. The cantor, accompanied by some other community members, traveled around to entertain the former camp prisoners. Nevertheless, the relatively small size of the community in comparison to the large numbers of newly arrived refugees gave the general impression that few people in the community were interested in helping them.

During these visits, it became apparent that only those few who hoped to find some close relative still alive in their countries of origin wanted to return home. The World Jewish Congress succeeded in persuading the Swedish government not to send back anyone against their will. After two months, the government offered the survivors the choice of returning to their countries of origin, immigrating to another country, or staying in Sweden. Those with surviving relatives left Sweden after the war, although reunion with parents or almost-forgotten relatives caused great emotional difficulties. Those who wanted to stay were given work permits for jobs that the Swedes themselves refused, such as household or factory work.

Before 1939, aid to refugees had been almost non-existent, but slowly increased every time new refugees were permitted into the country. The first refugees from Germany got no help from the government and only very little help from the Jewish community. The second group, arriving after 1944, received some help from the government and a little help from the Jewish community. Still later arrivals experienced the increased help the Swedish government was prepared to give, which ended up supporting the refugees on the same minimum standard of living that the Swedish population enjoyed.

SURVIVORS IN SWEDEN

The Swedish government took good care of the physical needs of the survivors. Medical care was excellent, and the people were provided with all the food they could eat, plus some pocket money. The pocket money was most often used to buy additional white bread, of which these once-starving people could never have their fill. A few weeks into the recovery period, the survivors wanted to be completely free and protested against the fence separating them from the outer world. They were reassured that the fences were there only to defend them from all the curious people who daily gathered around them. As soon as work permits were issued, the survivors left the camps and started to work.

The child survivors, those under the age of eighteen, were provided with educational opportunities. The Aliens Commission (*Utlanningskommissionen*), the organization empowered to decide on plans for the newcomers, organized boarding schools for them. These schools were situated all around the country, far from cities and distractions, and were run by teachers who, like their students, were survivors. The authorities did not interfere with the curricula, and thus the teachers were free to apply their own ideas. This resulted in great differences in the aim of the schools. Some of them gave a very formal and authoritarian education; others (like the Smedsbo school) used new democratic ideas to offer a more diversified education (as at Visingsö). All of them taught Jewish and Swedish matters, some (like Stratenbo) stressing the *chalutz* (Zionist pioneer) spirit and preparing the children for *aliyah* (immigration to Israel). Today, many of these children continue to live in kibbutzim in Israel.

PSYCHICAL NEEDS

The Swedes, both Jews and gentiles, tending to be of a cold nature, did not realize that the survivors were also in need of psychical support. Very few were invited by families to visit on a regular basis, and the longing for a family life resulted in hasty marriages, often to unsuitable partners. To begin with, the Swedes wanted to hear all about what happened in the different concentration camps, and the survivors obliged with their stories. However, the listeners could not really absorb the atrocities, and their nasty comments silenced the survivors. The majority of the concentration-camp survivors left Sweden within two to three years after their arrival. For the others, a period of lonely fighting started, a fight for adaptation, for a living, for a new identity, a new family, a new career. To achieve all this, they could not dwell on the past, on the bad memories. The Swedish Jews looked upon the newcomers with suspicion. The latter were mostly from Eastern Europe and although many of the earlier immigrants were from the same countries, they had assimilated. The Swedish Jews did not want to mix with the newcomers who looked different and spoke Yiddish. There was very little help to be had from the Jewish community, and the survivors did not feel understood by the staff, the non-Jewish social workers. Even today, there are survivors who continue to bear a grudge for the unfriendly welcome, remaining unwilling to join the community. Not many Jewish activities were available at that time, and hardly any possibilities for social get-togethers. The Jewish students occasionally arranged meetings for the young, but the older people had hardly any opportunities to meet Swedish Jews. For those staying in cities other than Stockholm, Göteborg, and Malmo, where Jews lived, there was not even the possibility of meeting other Jews. Some stayed in contact with the community in Stockholm and received intermittent visits from the cantor, but the difficulties involved in keeping a Jewish life discouraged most of them. In time, many married gentiles, assimilating completely.

THE SCHOOLS FOR THE CHILD SURVIVORS

Sara, born in 1930 in Hungary, came to the Smedsbo school after her recovery from TB. Many students still had not completely recovered, and after some time had to return to the sanatorium. Three years after having left the school, Sara wrote, "After a long trip by train, two other girls and I were heading by car towards the school. We passed through dark woods, and my thoughts circled around the sanatorium and the sickness I was leaving behind, and life and freedom ahead of me. What is the future going to be? Would I get disillusioned already at this first place, the school? The answer was no. From the first day, I felt at home there and I knew that I was going to like it also in the future."[4]

The children in the newly started boarding schools, having come directly from the concentration camps, could not understand the importance of going to school once again. "To begin with," remembered Sara, "I only saw a chaos of faces, noisy boys and girls, and after the quiet life at the sanatorium, this appeared to me as a very unusual picture. However, soon I adapted and I also became a regular 'Smedsboan.' "[5] Unlike Sara, some students were disillusioned and looked with great suspicion upon their teachers, the authority. They were reserved, very sensitive, and played a waiting game.

Eli Getreu and Ali Klein, the directors of Smedsbo, realized that the importance of the school was less to teach and more to imbue the children with an *elan de vivre*. Their work aimed to strengthen self-confidence, tolerance, and a sense of responsibility. Sara observed that "Once the teachers even helped a girl without any self-confidence to build up her personality. However, this was a single case, as the teachers had very little time for individual tutoring. As an excuse, it should be mentioned that the last six months before the end of the school, there were only two teachers to take care of fifty pupils."[6]

At first it seemed to Sara as if "everybody agreed on every topic with the teachers, but slowly I realized that real personalities were hiding behind the yelling youngsters."[7]

Getreu and Klein decided to apply the new democratic ideas represented by Neil's Summerhill school in England. In their free school, there was no coercion, no authoritarian rule. The rules were jointly decided upon by a board consisting of both teachers and pupils. The pupils monitored themselves and saw to it that the rules were respected. "In our childhood, all of us had been educated to accept the teacher as the highest authority and the biggest achievement of Smedsbo was that we are not any longer slaves to authority." Transgressors were taken care of by the pupil's own tribunal. The children were educated to think for themselves rather than to rely upon authorities, and the ambition of the teachers was to help the students find a meaning in life. "There is another issue around which Smedsbo achieved a lot," according to Sara. "After long discussions, sometimes with and sometimes without teachers present, we realized that besides Jews there are also other people in the world. Before we came to Smedsbo, we always thought and reacted from a Jewish point of view. It is only thanks to the school that we have become more internationally and humanistically oriented. For each of us, the school was very important, not primarily for our intellectual development, but mainly for the development of our opinions and outlook on life. I was far from being democratic before I came to Smedsbo and only there did I learn about democracy, women's liberation, free education, and so on."[8]

At Smedsbo, class attendance was voluntary, and at the beginning, nobody was compelled to study. Not too long after their arrival, lacking anything else to do, the children slowly decided to take part in the studies, and soon they followed the rules of the school. The language used was German and Hungarian, and the curriculum contained English and Hebrew, mathematics, religion, and child-rearing (a subject including sexual education). Discussions during classes were encouraged, and no marks were given.

Entertainment was provided in the evenings, including gramophone concerts, discourses, literary evenings, and discussions on different topics. Today, many survivors remember the time in these schools as their best time in Sweden. "One of my best memories from Smedsbo is my first Friday night at school. At seven o'clock, we gathered in one of the barracks to start celebrating the Sabbath. The pupils started by performing short sketches and dances. One dance was very pretty. A handcuffed woman dressed in black, seemingly in agony and pain, yearned for freedom. After a long struggle, she succeeded in getting loose. She got rid of her black gown and was transformed from a disfigured ghetto Jewess into a pioneer. I admired this woman tremendously and, for the first time, I felt togetherness with the Smedsboans. This feeling deepened still more during the evening when I and the other two newcomers also performed small pieces, trying to entertain the others, trying to show ourselves worthy to them."[9]

At the beginning, though, the youngsters had difficulties coping with the freedom at the school. After their concentration camp experience, in many cases preceded by an authoritarian upbringing, it took them some time to learn to live with freedom. The teachers could discern three phases of learning to live with freedom: the first being freedom as equal to chaos, resulting in disorientation; the second, freedom from commitments, resulting in unwillingness to accept rules; and finally, freedom with responsibility, resulting in independent individuals who take responsibility for themselves and their peers. During one meeting, the students discussed "some carpets to be moved from one room to the other. It was found that the carpets were not justly divided among the pupils and the discussion went on with great seriousness. I was impressed," revealed Sara, "and shaken at the same time, that the question of the carpets was talked about with the same zeal, seriousness, and accuracy as the world problems are discussed at the United Nations. At first, I supported it: a fellow citizen of Smedsbo had been wronged, and this had to be put right, even when it was only about a carpet."[10]

The age limit for attending these schools was eighteen years, and upon reaching their eighteenth birthday, they had to leave. However, before leaving, they were offered help to learn a trade and most also received state or community scholarships to continue their education. Sara "started school at the Birkagarden, the People's University in Stockholm. The studies take all my time," she said to an interviewer four years after she had left Smedsbo. She goes to the cinema or the theater only occasionally. "In a month, I will have finished my second year and at that time, I will have to have decided about my future what I want to become."

Unfortunately not all survivors under the age of eighteen had the privilege of going to school. Some immediately started to work in factories, even before these schools had been organized, and thus never discovered them. The schools were closed down in June 1948.

CHILD SURVIVORS FASHION ADULT LIVES

About one-third of those who arrived in 1945 stayed on in Sweden. Some of the students who had to leave the school, having reached the age of eighteen, had not completely recovered from TB and, therefore, were sent back to the sanatorium. This was the case for Sara. She stayed in different hospitals until 1950, embarking on higher education after two months of convalescence. At the time of the interview, her "highest wish is to be a social worker. The years in the different hospitals taught me a lot about the sick, and I would like to use my experiences to help others. If I cannot get the necessary education, I still hope to be able to work in a hospital."

Clara was fifteen when she was brought to Sweden on a stretcher with TB in both her lungs. She spent almost seven years in different sanatoria. After she was discharged, she took a course preparing her to become a laboratory assistant and then started working immediately. Clara has continued to work in a hospital, perhaps because she never felt completely recovered herself.

Other girls were given an opportunity to go to England. Because the Jewish population of Sweden was so small, the religious Jews both in Sweden and in the United States worried that the girls who had survived the camps would eventually marry gentiles. The fact that there were many more young women than men among the survivors added to this worry. Thus, an American organization, the Joint Distribution Committee, offered to help the Jewish community to give scholarships for studies in the Beth Jaakov school in London. As a consequence, quite a number of girls decided to become teachers there. Only a few, who had found out about surviving members of their family, returned to their countries of origin. The rest left for the United States, Australia, or Israel (until 1948, Palestine). In that regard, Sara was dissatisfied with the school's "continuous propaganda regarding Zionism." She understood "that this was necessary in a way; however, often it had the wrong effect. Nobody can tell us where to find happiness and what will suit the individual."[11] Years later, she expressed her own interest in living in Israel. "Sometime in the future, I would like to emigrate to Israel. I enjoy Sweden very much, but I cannot feel at home here. Once deracinated, it is difficult to grow new roots and I hope to be able to help build up a Jewish state."

For those who remained in Sweden, adaptation progressed slowly. The survivors stayed together most of the time and seldom mixed with the original Jewish population. In some cases, young girls were adopted by well-to-do families, but the emotional climate was so strange to them that they very seldom could feel a real sense of belonging. On the other hand, although no Swedish classes were available to foreigners, most of the newcomers learned the language quite quickly, and ultimately, adaptation to Swedish life went well. The political climate was very positive. On the surface, this was a democratic country with no visible antisemitism. The xenophobia that the newcomers experienced now and then was attributed to the isolated life the Swedes had led during the past centuries, and soon people learned to feel at home. Many of these new Swedes achieved satisfactory careers in science and commerce. The older survivors tended to take up trades, while the child survivors turned to higher education before starting their careers. Among the survivors and child survivors who enrich Swedish life today, there are well-known painters and writers, professors in research and medicine, musicians, and even a member of Parliament.

In their private lives, some young survivors attempted to cope with their need to belong by quickly finding a life-partner. Often they married without considering whether the match was suitable. Unhappy marriages resulting from these ill-considered decisions were not at all unusual.

Like many others, Clara's marriage unfortunately did not turn out well. In 1958 Clara had emigrated to Israel where she married a Romanian Jew. The couple had two girls. Clara reported that she stayed in the marriage only because of the children. The girls turned out to be very gifted and achieved professional careers. One became a medical doctor, the other an artist, but to Clara's great sorrow, they are still unmarried.

Sara had not married at the time of her interview. "All the time in the hospital, I have been waiting for the time when I shall be free and now I cannot handle my freedom." Nevertheless, during "these last few years I have been able to leave the hospital and live a private life. Now, my hope is in my future work and in the home I shall build. I am happy to have hope, it gives me joy. In all, I am happy about my life." Sara did marry. She remained in Sweden and married a gentile with whom she had one son. He became a physicist and gave Sara two grandchildren.

Isaac fell in love with a German woman at the age of thirty-one and moved to Germany. With the help of his wife, he started a restaurant there, which he successfully operated for twenty-five years. He had a son, whom he finds ungrateful and selfish. Unfortunately, his marriage broke up and he returned to Sweden.

AGING SURVIVORS

The trauma of the Holocaust was not forgotten. However, it was not until the early 1980s that the social workers of the Jewish community— many of them children of survivors—took notice and realized that, despite their seemingly normal lives, survivors were still burdened. Suppression or repression of their traumatic experiences did not free them. After a hectic professional life, these people, by now mostly retired and living alone, suffered from the long-term psychological effects of the atrocities they had experienced, but had never worked through. They displayed many of the emotional and physical symptoms of PTSD (posttraumatic stress disorder). More and more of the aging survivors complained of psychosomatic ailments. A case in point is Clara, who lives alone after her husband's death.

She is sickly and complains of various psychosomatic symptoms. She is disillusioned, has developed a depression, and has very poor relationships with
her daughters.

In the early 1990s many of the child survivors felt ready to confront their
suffering and to start to talk about their traumatic histories. The first child
survivor group did not start until 1993. After a short time, three distinct
subgroups crystallized, each with a different background and a different fate:
(1) children who arrived from Germany before the war; (2) those who were
in hiding; and (3) those who were in camps. Each set of survivors was
differently affected by their experiences. However, what remained in common was a reluctance to discuss the past and its effects upon the second
generation.[12]

WORKING THROUGH AND SOCIALIZING AT THE CAFÉ 84

In order to relieve the symptoms of the survivors, a Social Day Care
Center was established in Stockholm in 1984. This center, Café 84, was
named for the year it started, and has a unique program developed by the
author of this chapter. The center offers survivors a warm and accepting
meeting place, a forum that favors openness, and an atmosphere in which
they can be themselves.

The center's goal is to ease daily life, infuse courage, help members accept
life as it is, and, recognizing that traumas of this magnitude cannot be
healed, help them learn to live with the painful memories.

Café 84 is not just a self-help model. The center is led by a professional
psychologist who is a survivor. As a trained group facilitator and individual
psychotherapist, she is able to help survivors with their ongoing struggles
and to intervene in crisis situations. Members are allowed to move at their
own pace, to talk or not talk about their Holocaust experiences. The program provides members with the possibility of scrutinizing their own pasts
and coming to terms with them, while the psychologist focuses on the here-
and-now, taking a wait-and-see stance.

Some, like Isaac, complain that they have been silenced forever. Isaac
maintains he cannot open up because there was nobody to listen when he
wanted to talk about his experiences. He has told his wife hardly anything
and has said very little to his son. He says his life has been completely
destroyed.

Moreover, the second generation, the offspring of survivors, have not
been left unscathed. They feel the pain of their parents' wounds; they carry
invisible scars. Therefore, the center also allows members to review the relationships with their offspring in the light of other members' experiences.
Clearly, Clara, Isaac, Sara, and Jacob manifest vastly different capacities for
relationships. Clara, depressed and lonely, is not on good terms with her

children. Isaac, retired in Sweden, remains mute, bitter, and in poor health; he is critical of his son. Sara seems content in her family and at peace with herself as she continues to be active in her second vocation: She has become a writer. Jacob never talked about his war experiences except to his family. He told his children a little at a time, and now they know all about his life. He thinks that the children have been positively influenced by the fact that he always has been open with them. Only lately has he started to feel the need for communicating and sharing also with others.

The participants meet daily, between two and five in the afternoon, for discussions. These meetings are indirectly therapeutic, though no classical psychotherapy techniques are used. Members may choose the moments they are ready to talk and reveal themselves in the group. Some people schedule individual talks with the psychologist; however, the need for individual therapy seems to surface only in connection with acute current traumas. Generally, the elderly survivors feel that they have always managed their emotional difficulties without needing help. Thus, group members tend not to bring in current individual problems until a new loss occurs, which activates the earlier personal and Holocaust losses. Then, at long last, these may be looked at.

Other daily activities are also scheduled at the center, and the total program gradually helps the survivors. The activities include physical education—refreshing for the aching, elderly bodies and very much appreciated—led by a new Russian immigrant with knowledge of yoga-gymnastics; films with Jewish content, often in Yiddish; painting, under the leadership of a child survivor who became a professional artist; cinema; theater; and boat or bus excursions.

Every Friday evening at the Café 84, *Kabalath Shabbath* is celebrated with the lighting of candles, *kiddush*, and the blessing over *challah*. Refreshments are served and musical or other entertainment is provided. Those without families appreciate the center as the only place in Stockholm where they can celebrate the Sabbath communally. Attendance averages 60 to 70 people. Joyous holidays, such as Chanukkah and Purim and members' birthdays, as well as the anniversary of the opening of Café 84, are celebrated. Once yearly, participants may also avail themselves of a ten-day stay at the Jewish summer camp, Glämsta.

Participation in Café 84 has changed the lives of many survivors. They have noticed improvements in their spirit, their sleep, and even in their health. Their children concur and also noticed that their parents have become less dependent. Survivors often state that the center is their second home. Indeed, there was a need for it when they arrived in Sweden, and some complain that had it not started so late, it might have prevented some of the ailments they suffer from today.

The Legacy of Survivors

The settling of the Holocaust survivors in Sweden resulted in a very active Jewish life. Today's Jewish population in Sweden numbers about 17,000, mostly clustered in the big cities—Stockholm, Göteborg, and Malmo. A Jewish center flourishes in Stockholm. There is the Hillel School for pupils aged up to thirteen, and special Jewish curricula within one of the Swedish schools, Ahlstromska, for ages thirteen to sixteen. Glämsta Summercamp for children, a Jewish theater, a Jewish service house for the aged and the sick, and the Social Day Care Center for survivors, Café 84, are all signs of a thriving Jewish community.

NOTES

1. This unpublished poem was written in 1952 by Eva Löwenthal, a woman of Hungarian origin married to a German Jew. It expresses her sense of loss, dislocation, and identity confusion.

2. It turned out that after some time hiding with the partisans, Jacob's father had also been caught. Miraculously, at the time of liberation, the father happened to be in the same camp as the rest of the family, and thus they were reunited. The family returned to their former home, but after some time, the father decided to leave for Sweden to join a surviving brother. The family moved in with the brother, and the parents started to work in a factory.

3. As a child during the war, before their incarceration in 1942, Jacob lived with his family in the ghetto of Lodz. Soon his father disappeared to join the partisans, leaving the mother alone with the child. When all children under the age of ten were to be taken on a transport, his mother obtained a false work permit for him, stating his age to be ten years. He "worked" as an errand boy in the factory, but in 1942, both he and his mother were taken to a concentration camp.

4. Eli Getreu, "Practical Pedagogy in a Boarding School: Experiences from Work with Youngsters Liberated from Concentration Camps" (author's translation), in *Pedagogisk Tidskrift* 80, no. 3–6 (1952): 39–126.

5. Ibid.
6. Ibid.
7. Ibid.
8. Ibid.
9. Ibid.
10. Ibid.
11. Ibid.

12. Ingrid Lomfors, "The Jewish Refugee Children from Nazi Germany" (Unpublished doctoral dissertation, University of Gottenburg, 1996). According to Lomfors, the younger the survivors were, the more easily they adapted; the older they were, the guiltier they felt for surviving their parents who had been killed. Their surroundings increased these feelings, telling them to be grateful for the food and shelter they got. Lomfors found no differences between the children brought up in the camps and those in Jewish or non-Jewish families. Most of them have tried hard and succeeded in assimilating the Swedish life. They have become Swedish.

All had been silent about their background, and to this day, only a few have volunteered to talk. Lomfors advances as a reason for the survivors' silence: Those who were not concentration camp inmates might have compared their own fate with the lot of those who were in camps, concluding that their own fate had been so much easier, they might have believed they have nothing to tell. However, this author is of the opinion that, while striving towards adaptation, the survivors remained silent to hide their Jewish origin. Today, more and more of them feel old memories awaken, and many more volunteer to talk.

15

History of the Australian Child Survivor Groups: Melbourne and Sydney

Paul Valent and Litzi Hart

MELBOURNE

Paul Valent

The Melbourne Child Survivor group came into being in February 1990.

At the 1989 International Society of Traumatic Stress Studies, Sarah Moskovitz casually asked me whether I was a child survivor and whether I would attend her workshop. "No." I replied, "My parents were survivors." "Where were you during the war?" she wanted to know. "In Hungary." "How old were you at the end of the war?" she pressed on. "Seven." "So you are a child survivor," she concluded. Still objecting, I explained that "I was not in a concentration camp."

"You are a child survivor." As such I attended her workshop.

At the end of the workshop I met Ervin Staub who is my age and also had been in Budapest during the war. We talked for days like two Martians discovering each other. I sought out other Martians in Melbourne. The release from my world of strange grayness into one of solid recognition had begun. I felt that others should have the opportunity for this to happen to them, too.

With that in mind, I contacted Litzi Hart, who had already formed a Sydney group. Helen Gardner, from the Jewish Crisis Center, and I advertised, and we gathered thirty people to our first meeting. We went around the room, many introducing their true identities for the first time. Litzi, who had come down to us by bus from Sydney, set the tone with her simplicity. We heard a child survivor telling her story for the first time. Then we talked. For some, this was their first-ever group where they felt at home. They wanted to join. We decided to meet on the same Sunday of the next month and subsequent months. We have been meeting on the first Sunday of each month regularly for nearly eight years.[1]

What should we do once we were together was the big question. Oh, we must not look at our navels and be self-absorbed in the past—but what is the point of being just like any other Jewish group having film nights and collecting money for Israel? What distinguishes us? Well, Litzi had inspired us with her story, and many started to tell parts of their own. Shall some of us tell our stories? And let us record them? It was decided: We would tell our stories. And videotape them? And we did.

But two a night was too much. It would not leave time to go into details. So after two attempts, only one person has been scheduled to present at each meeting. We have lived through and recorded almost thirty stories now, and they are in our library and in the Yad Vashem archives. One person tells his or her story, but it is always *our* stories that are told, too—from different angles. We have continued to have twenty to thirty at each meeting, though our membership list has grown to 200.

All child survivors are welcome to our meeting from wherever in the world they may come. We meet at the Holocaust Center at 7:30 on the first Sunday of the month. Well, we start a little late. Then we make our announcements. New attendees introduce themselves. Then, for a little over an hour, one member of our group tells his or her story. The stories are from the heart, not from paper; and they include the whole life, not only the war years. Family members have attended also, and at times they contribute to the person's story. How much to tell? This is not therapy, and some things are difficult to tell a group, but we are honest and we expose ourselves, for we trust each other. The video? Yes, we want the world to truly know what happened to us children.

We break for coffee for half an hour. New people, who had not seen other child survivors since adolescence and had not realized they were child survivors, catch up with each other. People who had similar experiences compare notes. Then we go back and ask questions. How did you feel when the machine gun was pointed at you? Why was there more anger with the Jews in charge than the Germans? Forbidden feelings are explored for the first time. Why did your mother not want to listen to how you were affected, and how did this feel for you?

And then we move on to issues. What happened to our memories? What happened to traumatic memories altogether? With all you experienced, why did you not cry? Why do we not cry? What happened to our emotions in those times—and since? And love? Yes, what happens to emotions altogether? Oh, the anguish that we were brave enough to explore recently—not to be able to love our children as we would wish! We are very kind and nonjudgmental with each other, for we always see the persecuted child. And we also remember all we have survived: Such awful things happened to us.

And in spite of that, we have achieved. But no, we are not unscathed by any means. Yet we do love as best we can, and we are nice children beneath it all. At the end of the meetings, we sort of hug each other mentally, and we feel just a little wiser.

At times we had experiential workshops instead of stories. In them we explored specific feelings such as abandonment and shame. And then again, we ask ourselves: Do we need this? Shouldn't we rather look to the future, help other children, help the Holocaust Center, educate the world? People oscillate in their explorations and sharing. Similarly, some come and go, and may return after a long time. But we persevere in our different ways. I have learned that this is exactly what people like us must do: remember, then have a break—the same way as quite a few of us have now been back to the places of persecution and then returned to Australia. There and back and there again, often—both geographically and in the mind.

In the group schedule as well, we have taken breaks to do things other than looking into our pasts. Each December we have a social occasion at a member's place. Occasionally we get together with the other generations of survivors to hear a visitor or to commemorate special events.

On the Tuesdays following our meetings, the committee meets at one of our homes to review the last event and prepare future ones, keeping the desires of the members in mind. We have developed a solid core of committee members and have become such friends—we can say anything to each other—like a group of friends we could not have in our youth.

The Melbourne group has participated in some conferences and, goodness, have we hosted a couple! But first, in January 1991, some of us went to a conference in Sydney and again Sarah (Moskovitz) was there. We were surprised to find that we child survivors in the two cities were so similar! Not only the Melbourne and Sydney group members were similar. Those of us who attended The Hidden Child Conference in New York, in May 1991, realized that we child survivors are like siblings, no matter from where in the wide world we came.

In preparation for The Hidden Child Conference we had started to inform the local communities of Australia about who we were. But now we came out in front of the whole world! Richard Rozen came out of the cupboard, as it were, where he had hidden for thirteen months as a child; he was all over the newspapers in the United States, and his story came to be printed in two books. I also came out of hiding in very good company indeed, when I presented a paper while on a panel with Sarah Moskovitz, Judith S. Kestenberg, and Robert Krell. I have given papers in Amsterdam at an international Traumatic Stress Society meeting, and I was proud to represent the Australian Child Survivors in Jerusalem. I have written and presented a number of papers, and have written a book, *Child Survivors: Adults Living with Childhood Trauma*. I mention these activities because they are part and product of our group as a whole. Through my experience,

I have realized that we child survivors not only have a unique historical significance, but also a unique psychological significance for victims and survivors of all kinds. In our group, we feel that our experiences must be shared to help many others in the world.

We hosted an International Child Survivor conference in January 1993. The theme was "Last Witnesses to the Holocaust," because by then we understood our special historical significance. The program included Sarah Moskovitz as our keynote speaker, plenaries with rescuers, a three-generation survivor family, and workshops ranging from "I Never Said Goodbye," "Loss of Childhood and Impact on Parenting," "Learning to Trust; Feeling Safe," to "Physical and Sexual Abuse of Children." It was a marvelous conference, with a persistent glow.

In July 1994, Dr. Judith S. Kestenberg visited the child survivor groups in Melbourne and Sydney, and Melbourne organized a conference around her visit. In addition to her lecture, we scheduled three-generational workshops: child survivors, adult survivors, and children of survivors—we talked with each other, our parents, and our children. In many instances we spoke and listened properly for the first time. This conference, too, was very successful.

Dr. Kestenberg not only interviewed many of our group members, but also gave our fledgling interview group a fillip: The group is now part of the interviewing group of the International Study of Organized Persecution of Children. And so we have played host to our mothers, Sarah and Judith, and are pleased to be able to carry on their work. We are so grateful that we had a chance to say "thank you" to them, *en famille*.

Slowly we are beginning to look outside our Melbourne Child Survivor Group and to become involved in a number of areas. We are close to our Sydney group and feel close (albeit for many of us in a vague way) to other child survivor groups around the world. We moved from the Jewish Crisis Center to the Holocaust Museum in 1991 and, since then, have had close links with the adult survivor group. Some of us work for the museum and are guides there. We are proud of the Second Generation Group, which hived off from us and is now a very viable group with close links to our own. We partake in many transgenerational functions, for instance in the Fiftieth Year of Liberation celebrations and the annual commemorations. At the same time, we are pleased that we are not beholden to any other group, nor are we split between hidden and non-hidden children. We are child survivors. That is who we are.

As participating members of the Child Survivor Group, we have become more confident and proud of who we are. We reach out to other groups, remembering the many child survivors who may still be in hiding. We send our newsletter regularly to all who have been to our group, even to those who attended only once, and to those who have expressed interest in the group but have not yet made it to a meeting. Sometimes such people come after a year or two, when they are ready. We want them to know they belong to us all the time. Some are ambivalent about exposing who they are, others have too much pain, and others still maintain they are far from pain. They are the same as the child survivors attending meetings, only a little more scared.

When we look back over the last eight years, we see how greatly things have changed. We are a viable group. We know ourselves and people know us. Our voices are heard; even in the community at large, they know who we are. We have an identity, a very respectable one. We have a voice. We have a history, from the past to the future. Our individual members have come a long way, too, in their quest to know themselves, and we have a better idea of the meaning of what happened to us. Of course, things are not rosy. What happened to us was horrible, and knowing it better is not a delight. But, as a result of our group experience, we are a little more in control and can help others a little more. We have triumphed through our survival—unfortunately not all of us, and not completely, so we grieve as we celebrate, too.

What of the future? We know that soon we will be the last survivors. Like all children, we need to grow into our roles, and we feel that these should not be prescribed for us. We have deep respect for our parents, the adult survivors, and for their memories as well as for our own. For the moment, we still need to define ourselves further and to find deeper meanings and purposes in the way we have been shaped. In the meantime, we are pleased that we can do so together, and together appreciate our lives as survivors. We are pleased to join hands with you and to share with you.

SYDNEY

Litzi Hart

The Sydney Child Survivors Group began in 1986. The seeds were sown in 1985, at the Forty-Fifth Anniversary of the Holocaust, during a week-long gathering of Holocaust survivors with guest speakers from other countries.[2] I was in the audience listening to Sarah Moskovitz tell my story. Telling Sarah had been the first time I had told anyone everything I remember. Eighteen months later, Sarah came back to Australia. We then had a gathering of survivors (mostly child survivors, some older) and spouses. As a result, we agreed to meet and just to talk together over a cup of coffee in a private home. There were twenty of us, and we each told our story.

All this had been instigated by Sarah Moskovitz through Eva Engel, who is not a survivor, but feels like one. She talked, nudged us, cajoled, helped, and supported us. "Do it," she said. "We need it," she said. We were hesitant. It was so new, facing our past and other survivors for the first time. Then we did it! We were adults who had once been children in hiding, or in concentration camps, or traveling around on false papers. Our first meeting was at the Bnai Brith Lodge. There were twenty-five of us, all born after 1928. We had come to share experiences, to discuss a lot we had in common, to feel comfortable with each other, and to be acknowledged. A growing membership created a newsletter to keep in contact with one another and with those who didn't come to meetings—except now and again.

During our first year, six child survivors lit the six memorial candles at the Holocaust Commemoration Service. I gave my first speech in public. I told of meeting with old friends from youth-group days through the survivor group. We hadn't known about our common past. Nobody had talked before then. Not like now.

The group continued to meet in each other's homes, always with food and drinks. It was a stressful time for some; liberating for most. We wanted to be autonomous, though under the umbrella of the Association of Holocaust Survivors. Conflict! We tried to do things together, but they were not pleased. We needed to grow on our own, to develop by ourselves. Perhaps we would join later when we "grew up." We were not ready to get involved or to be organized, official, or to take responsibility; and some of us didn't want to "carry the burden of the Holocaust." We just wanted to be together and talk. And so we "separated" from the association and stopped trying to please them.

During the group meetings we told our stories. Some stopped coming, new people came, and we continued to grow. We were ready to do something other than talk. In 1989 we organized an International Jewish Cabaret. An evening of Hebrew, Russian, Yiddish, and English singing and dancing and music played to a full house. The community supported us, and close to $6,000 were presented to Kibbutz L'Ochamei Hagetaot for Project Yad Le Yeled (a memorial museum in Israel) in remembrance of the 150,000 children who died in the Holocaust—close to our hearts.

With the help of Sarah Moskovitz we made contact with the Los Angeles Child Survivors. They sent us their newsletter, we sent them our more modest one. Some of us went to the International Child Survivor Conference in California in 1990. Two hundred child survivors from all over the world gathered—all talking together, attending workshops, sharing meals, and socializing between. Fourteen people who had been interviewed by Sarah for her book, *Love Despite Hate*, were there. Meeting them again, I met my childhood past. Later, we made connections with New York, Canadian, French, and British child survivors.

Then came a phone call out of the blue: "My name is Paul Valent. Sarah Moskovitz gave me your name, and I'd like to start a child survivor group in Melbourne." I told him about our group, and in February 1990, the Melbourne group was formed.

We continued to meet every six weeks or so in Sydney. The questions "What is our aim? Where are we going?" popped up every so often. Meanwhile, we wanted Sarah Moskovitz to meet our expanding group. Why not have a conference? Sarah would be the guest speaker. How to pay for this? Once again we had help from the community, though mainly we helped ourselves by organizing a fundraising dinner. In January 1991, the conference had became a reality. Five Melbourne child survivors came to our workshops, with lunch, dinner, music, and fun included. We gathered more survivors, and it brought us closer together.

In January 1992, twenty Sydney child survivors went to the Melbourne Child Survivor Conference. It was marvelous, exciting, stimulating, and well organized. New friends were talking, listening, and revealing themselves in an atmosphere of safety. We were maturing and becoming "doers" as well as "talkers."

Our meetings continue, but we are now too large a group to meet in members' homes, and go instead to the Folk Centre, a communal center for the aged. We still have questions: Should we be structured? Should we have a constitution? Should we join the Board of Deputies? We have a committee and more people want to be involved. Although we now have energy enough driving us, we want to remain informal and apolitical.

We have become more involved with the community as individuals. Sydney now has a wonderful Jewish Museum where many of us are "historians." We feel the need to give visitors who come to learn about the Holocaust a first-hand account, to tell our own stories. We collaborate with the older survivors in this. They approached us, presenting their need to have us continue their work. We will be the last survivors. We know that.

Next year (1995) is the fiftieth anniversary of liberation. "Would we join the planning committee," the adult survivors wanted to know, "to plan the dinner together with the descendants and the older survivors?" Perhaps we are ready to take responsibility. We are being acknowledged. Meanwhile, we continue meeting with each other, and we remain unstructured, though we have a committee and disseminate information through our newsletter. At the Jewish Museum we guide, help launch books, and generally involve ourselves more with the community, while continuing to be part of the growing emergence of child survivors all over the world.

NOTES

1. 1989 to 1994 and continuing.
2. People like Yaffa Eliach and Sarah Moskovitz who spoke about the children from Terezin who went to Winkfield House, Surrey, England.

16

Trauma: A View from the German Side

Charlotte Kahn

"You know, I'm like everybody else on the planet: I am deeply struck
by the suffering of my own. It's a terrible truth that identity is steeped
in the blood of martyrs, a phenomenon you can see clear round the
world. . . . The Armenians, the Kurds. The Igbo. The Rom. The list is
damn near endless."[1]

—Scott Turow

INTRODUCTION

This chapter will address the struggles of some non-Jewish German children
with their World War II past. ("Non-Jewish German" may seem to be re-
dundant to those unaware that, prior to 1933, Jews had been full-fledged
German citizens of Jewish faith. It was no different than in the United States
today, where citizenship is independent of religion or of race.) To present
a vivid picture of the children's few pleasures and many trials, whenever
possible some of their stories will be recounted in their own—now adult—
words.[2]

During interviews focused on their childhood and adolescent experiences
in Nazi Germany, almost all of those questioned told of disrupted school
careers, due first to the closing of Catholic and progressive schools, and later
to their conscription into the work force and the army. They suffered dislocation, dispersal, air raids, and loss of family members on the battlefield
as well as at home. Many were strafed by the Allied air forces, as they fled
on foot from the feared Russian troops advancing westward. The postwar
period was punctuated by intense hunger.

While these youngsters' experiences were not comparable to Jewish children's incarceration in concentration and extermination camps, nor their
work and hunger and uprootedness comparable to forced labor, starvation,

and emigration, I believe we should not ignore them. The oldest interviewees were young teenagers, only thirteen in 1933, at the official onset of the Nazi regime; the youngest were thirteen in 1945, at the end of World War II. They reported the events simply as happenings in children's lives.

Originally I conducted these interviews out of curiosity about the psychic and material conditions of my former German playmates and classmates.[3] What did they think about the occurrences around them, and what became of them after I emigrated? And what are their views about Hitler, Jews, and the Holocaust, in retrospect? Now I have other questions: Were the German children—and I—overprotected? Shielded from reality? Were we naïve children at an age when today's youth are sophisticated?

Can we believe the interviewees? Is it really true that most did not know until after the war about deportations, forced labor, and extermination?[4] Was it age-appropriate, perhaps, that they did not grasp the larger picture, focusing instead on daily, dissociated events in their lives?

For the purposes of this anthology, the most important questions are: What were the sequelae to their experiences? and, How did they cope?

THE INVESTIGATION

Between 1988 and 1992 I interviewed nearly one hundred individuals born between 1920 and 1933. Of these, most of the fifty-three formerly West Germans met in small groups and some were seen individually in 1988. In January 1992 twenty more people were interviewed individually in the West. In the East, twenty people were interviewed in 1990, and some of them for a second time one year later, after the Berlin Wall had come down. In East Germany, group meetings were impossible—people did not dare speak up except in absolute privacy.[5]

All but the 1992 interviewees were self-selected in response to newspaper announcements of the project. Because the announcement in December 1991 had but two respondents (probably due to the holiday and vacation schedules), a helpful Protestant clergyman called his parishioners, who eagerly participated. (Incidentally, this minister had been instrumental in building a memorial chapel in Duisburg, am Rhein, on the site of that city's erstwhile synagogue, consumed by the *Kristallnacht* [Night of Broken Glass] fire.) In the East, the selection of participants was further limited by the fact that not all respondents had telephones, and only those who could be called were contacted to arrange interview appointments.

The consistency of the testimony lends confidence in the validity of the reports, despite the inconsistently selected (research sample) population. The reports were consistent regarding the accounts of air raids and of evacuations; the interviewees' awareness of the fate of Jews, concentration camps, and deportations; their experiences in the various youth organizations; in their political awareness; and their wartime work assignments. Men and women alike reported having witnessed or heard about Russian soldiers raping German girls and women. "We had great fear of the Russians, who had three days' *liberty of the victor* [during which] they were allowed to rape, destroy and plunder everything." Regarding the Americans, "they didn't force themselves into the houses to rape the girls. They only took them when they were alone with them somewhere."

Selected interview statements, organized according to the topics of air raids, Jews, youth organizations, and political awareness, will be presented here. Following this material, a discussion will focus on the coping abilities of traumatized children and youths.

AIR RAIDS

Frieda, who had been assigned to a rescue squad, was sent to the site of a train that had been attacked. Every passenger had sustained head shots. Not one was alive. With the other teenagers on the squad, she had to carry out the dead.

Wilma witnessed an attack on a passenger train under somewhat different circumstances. She was on her way to visit her grandmother in Schlesien when the train was attacked by aerial dive bombers. The train stopped. "Someone grabbed me and pulled me away" under the train. "There were dead [people] there, but I didn't register it as a child. My only concern was to get back onto the train before it pulled out. I was happy to be inside."

Gerd, who was ninety kilometers away from Dresden at the time of the big bombing, remembers: "It was as if a volcano had erupted. There were refugees from Czechoslovakia and Schlesien who were in camps, in tents. People were barred from the city because of the danger of epidemics. The corpses were lined up at the railroad tracks."

Heinz recalls an air raid in Essen, one day before his twelfth birthday. "Everything was burning. People were burning . . . it was unimaginable." He paused, perhaps reliving the experience. Then he continued, "And one gets so immensely upset." Again he paused before going on. "I can still see myself running through the burning street, not looking right or left, only to get to a shelter. And then I had to take care of many little children in this shelter because the grownups all went out to save whatever could be saved. So I had a horde of kids all night long. I was still young myself."

Edith was interred under rubble during a bombing. Many people around her in the basement shelter died, including her mother, sister, grandmother, and neighbors. Her father was at the front. After sixteen hours she was excavated, then hospitalized for weeks with broken bones; she was sick for months. She recounted, "I returned to Berlin in a hospital train."

Inge "no longer had anything to wear" after an air raid. "We were practically naked as we were brought out from the burning cellar . . . the end of 1944. I received a pair of sandals . . . and a pair of men's slacks."

YOUTH, GROUP-LIFE, POLITICAL AWARENESS

Heinz, minding the little ones in the shelter, had to take on adult responsibilities too soon.[6]

Emil, born in Italy of German parents, also reported resentfully, "Our youth was stolen from us [by the war]. . . . Nowadays the youth flips out at fifteen; I flipped out (*ausgeflipt*) at twenty-five, after I finished my [interrupted] preparatory schooling."

Winfried thinks "others still do not believe that the *Jungvolk* (a section of the Hilter Youth) was quite easygoing." His experience was that "the premilitaristic training aspects have been immeasurably exaggerated." He was horrified by a book he saw that painted a picture as if "all that ever happened were marches and parades." According to him, it was not like that. For many other boys and girls it was not like that.

Helmut was aware that he had much fun in the *Fliegerhitlerjugend* (aviation Hitler-youth), where the boys built "glider planes . . . used for . . . [their] first flights." They spent weekends flying. "Nevertheless," said Helmut, "it served the military insofar as we had some pretraining."

Ursula, a West German interviewee, sees that her children are starved for information and, she says, "we can be of more help, because, thank God, we do not have to justify ourselves. Others, older, build a defensive wall, because they don't want to have been the [bad] ones." As a child, she continued, German children knew only what a *KZ* (pronounced *kaahtset*, for *Konzentrationslager*, which means concentration camp) is, "that it exists," but not what happens there. On the night train to Prague (where she was sent on evacuation) "little girls told jokes [and] someone said, 'Shh, quiet, or you'll go to the *KZ*.' "

Erich, who attended boarding school, explained that he spent too little time at home to know his parents' attitudes.[7]

Ursula remembered discussions about the annexation of Austria and the Sudetenland, but not of "German internal politics."

Marte was unaware at the time that it was Hitler who started the war. For her it was a pleasure to be in *Kinderlandverschickung* (children's evacuation of school classes) and afterward in the *BDM* (*Bund Deutscher Mädel*, League of German Girls). She found it great being organized and living in a community. Singing and marching was marvelous. She summed up with, "I thought it was nice that people watched us [marching . . . and] I hadn't a single political thought. I couldn't have had. . . . Unconsciously I was in a political compulsion."

Ninnette's home experience gave her a fuller perspective. She recounts, "I was the oldest by several years, so my father and I had our political conversations in the cellar. . . . in the cauldron [the washtub], we had hidden a [short-wave] radio—punishable by death. My father always said to me that you have to create a picture for yourself, based on both sides. [Therefore] we also listened to the German sender [as well as the British Broad-casting Corporation], because no newscast is objective. That impressed me, even influences my current thinking. [However, actually] to do anything was impossible. My father was already punished vocationally . . . because we were not in the Party." Even saying anything was unthinkable inasmuch as sometimes saying the manifest truth was interpreted as disloyalty. For ex-ample, after an air raid, Nanette's mother commented to a neighbor that " 'All of Karlsruhe is aflame.' 'What did you say? All of Karlsruhe is aflame?' 'Yes,' replied mother, 'take a look, from left to right, as far as I can see.' The neighbor replied, 'If you spread such news again, I'll bring you to where you belong!','' a threat to report the mother to the authorities, who would incarcerate her in a concentration camp.

Similarly *and* in contrast, one interviewee related that she had voiced her opinion at *home* that Germany could not emerge victorious against the com-bined powers of the United States, England, France, and the Soviet Union. Soon thereafter, she was called to an interrogation at the police headquar-ters. Although she stopped short of openly accusing her mother of betraying her, the use of a "testing the limits" method toward the end of the interview left not much doubt about who had turned her in. Only the intervention of her boss at work saved her from incarceration. It is general knowledge that in their patriotic fervor citizens betrayed each other, and that some children had been so indoctrinated they turned in their parents. However, this incident of a mother turning in her own child was a sad, almost un-believable story.

AWARENESS OF JEWS, CONCENTRATION CAMPS, DEPORTATIONS

Albert, born in 1927, remembers that he hadn't become aware of the fate of the Jews. *"Ist mir nicht so bewußt geworden"* ("It didn't become so con-scious for me") were his words. He never had had a pal or a classmate of Jewish origin. "Only through my father I once heard, [someone] had to walk around with the Yellow Star. We [children] saw the Star and didn't give it a thought. My father got very upset. He said, 'even those who earned the Iron Cross in World War I, [that is] those who also had fought for Germany . . . still had to walk around with that star.' [But] as children we were perhaps too young [to understand]."

Meinhard also said, "At the time I heard people speaking [about the Jews who had left], but I didn't give it any thought. [Only] in retrospect, I thought about it."

Herta said that, in contrast to today, at fourteen she with her marbles was still treated like a child. Her classmate, who had moved into the village, said that where she used to live, it smelled of burning human flesh. "That can't be," Herta said, "because then human beings would have to be

burned." Naïve and surprised, she immediately told her mother, who became agitated and frightened, and told her never to speak about that again.
That it could be reality never occurred to her. "It sounds so daft," she said.
"I have talked seriously with my daughter about that" because her daughter
told her, "You couldn't have lived through that time, when so much happened, and not noticed anything."

Maria knew of only one Jew, Mr. Guldowski, in whose business her
mother had worked beginning with an apprenticeship at age fourteen.
"*Mutti* (mother) cried. Because she started there as a quiet, thin, young
girl, [Guldowski] included her a little in the family. . . . Often she could
take things [foodstuffs] home, first into her parents' home, then [again]
when she was married. . . . We didn't have much. Father was unemployed.
. . . Then—it was surely 1938 . . . that mother came home . . . [when] the
ancient Oma (the Guldowski grandmother) died. And then Guldowski was
taken away and then the one daughter, with whom mother was sort of
friendly. . . . *Och*, I found that sad. . . . Mutti was so very sad when they
took away the Guldowskis . . . and somewhere that touched me too. . . . I
didn't know the old Guldowski, but that my Mutti was so touched, made
me feel uncomfortable. I felt sorry for her. . . . She cried so much."

Marte had thought people incarcerated in the *KZ* were criminals. She
believed it a good thing to have a fence between them and her. After the
war, while Marte (then sixteen) was in Czechoslovakia, she was part of a
group taken (by the Americans) to a place in the forest where ninety-nine
people had been shot and buried in a shallow mass grave. She said, "We
had to help dig up these people. They were already decomposing after weeks
of lying there. It was fiendishly difficult work . . . terrible. . . . The bodies
were put into gray, banana-shaped containers, loaded on a truck and taken
to a regular mass grave. . . . Then we were told these had been *KZ* inmates.
. . . I hadn't known anything of what had been happening around me."

Lore was also naive—until 1945, when she came to Schlesien to work in
a motor-vehicle office. The office was "on street level and I looked out
toward the back. And there I sometimes thought, 'for God's sake, what's
happening here?' There were the *Hiwis (Hilfswillige*, volunteer helpers).
They were brought from Russia, from Poland, from everywhere. . . . [In
these] munition factories . . . all night one could hear the motors running.
And there I saw how they beat up these young people terribly. . . . Where
my grandmother lived, when we looked out of the back window, there was
a sort of farm . . . and in the background was a camp, barracks . . . and there
one could sometimes hear the people screaming. . . . Everything had been
taken from them. . . . Summer and winter they had to go barefoot or they
wrapped rags around their feet. They were driven to the workplace like a
herd of sheep accompanied by [guards with] rifles and bayonets. . . . People
talked about it; not everyone thought it was a good thing; [but] no one

dared express opinions, because they thought, 'then you, yourself will wind up in such a camp.' "

Rita's story is an example of this: "I was employed by the City (Karlsruhe) and had to take the trolley at about seven in the morning to the *Marktplatz* [Marketplace]. There, I saw from the trolley that a synagogue was burning. . . . As I descended, I saw a tiny old man with a long beard pulling a little rack-wagon in which sat his wife, crying. Judging by their attire, they were the poorest—either a rag seller or someone from the old part of town with a pawnshop—about seventy years old. The man shuffled and dragged his feet. I asked whether I could help, asked where they were going. . . . He said, 'We are Jews and we have to go to the *Kleine Kirche* (Little Church).' I said, 'I will pull your wagon.' Then a uniformed man came along and shouted, 'What are you doing here? Are you also a Jew-pig? Get away from here or you'll also go where they belong!' I said 'But I can help take them there.' Thereupon he struck me with a stick so hard that I had to let go and run away." Yet, the real danger of winding up in a concentration camp did not deter everyone from doing something.

Frieda found out what her mother had done in 1938 *after* the war—not during the Nazi reign when children might inadvertently or deliberately betray their parents. Mother was standing near the window of their street-level apartment when Mr. Gold, chairman of the Jewish congregation passed by. He was being taken away. Mother thought, "My God, what will happen to the wife with her five little children?" That evening she heard something in the hall. She went to look and found Frau Gold and her children crouching in the corner near the cellar door. "What are you doing here?" asked Frieda's mother. Frau Gold was afraid for her children, afraid of being taken away. (Polish Jews were rounded up and sent back to the border of Poland several weeks before *Kristallnacht*.) At that point, Frieda's mother took another tenant into her confidence, a mother of seven, and the two set up air-raid shelter cots in the basement for the Gold family. Frieda's apartment was right above the cellar, and her mother told Mrs. Gold that in case people were going into the cellar for anything, she would warn her by stomping on the floor so she could quiet the children. Later, as a favor to the other tenants—many of whom thought the cellar was eerie—mother offered to go to the cellar for them to bring down or fetch any items like potatoes or coal. At the same time, she knocked twice at Mrs. Gold's door and left some things for her. Some weeks had passed when four *SS* men (storm troopers) came to the door, accusing Frieda's mother of hiding someone. Mother displayed her *Mutterkreuz* (Badge of Honor for mothering five children for Hitler and the Fatherland), called her accomplice as a witness, and challenged the *SS* men to prove their allegations. When the *SS* wanted to search the cellar, mother agreed and opened the door to the room where the gas meters hung. Because the doors opened in opposite directions, they concealed the center door to the room where the Golds were hiding. One of the men guarded mother, while the other three walked about with flash-lights, looking behind all the many items stored by the tenement inhabi-tants. In the end the *SS* were annoyed. Said one, "*Ja*, that's outrageous to send us here—as if these mothers of large families would risk their lives like that!" About one week after the search, a letter was dropped off. It said, "Please don't lock up [the entrance door] tonight," signed, *Rotes Mützchen* (Little Red Cap). Around half past ten that night, a large black car pulled up, someone with a cape and a big hat pulled down over the face got out, walked into the house, and before long, Frau Gold with her five children got into the car. They drove off. Mother said, "Thank God." Soon a post-card arrived. It said, "Forgot the little red cap, but even without the cap arrived safely." After the war, when food was scarce in Germany, many care packages arrived from Seattle without a return address, only "Regards, Red Cap."

DISLOCATION

During the interviews I often wondered how, even as adults, so many Germans could fail to make certain connections. Neither East nor West Germans related the Allied attack on Dresden to the German bombing of Coventry, for example. And I wonder whether the similarity—between the Nazis forcing all Jews to wear the identifying yellow Star of David and deporting them to ghettos and concentration camps, and the Poles insisting after the war that the Germans in the Polish territories wear an identifying arm band, and then deporting them in cattle cars or on foot—really escapes them. The use of some terminology indicates that at least unconsciously certain relationships were dimly perceived.

Louise reported indignantly, "The Poles treated us very badly . . . [T]hey tortured us [and soldiers] chased us out of apartments we had just made somewhat livable. . . . Every four weeks or so, we had to vacate our apart-ments. . . . Several times we were assaulted on the street, thrown into the ditch . . . and one day, in December 1946, I believe, it was selection." (Se-lection was the word used to decide who would live and who would die in the concentration camps.) Louise refers here to the population exchange and explains: "All the Germans were stuck into a freight train. . . . These cattle cars . . . were jammed full until no one else could fit and then [they were] sealed. [The train] was sent to the West. That was the *Vertreibung*—the banishment, expulsion, deportation. The railroad cars were sealed. We didn't know where [the train] was going. I don't know how long we trav-eled—one week, a fortnight. . . . Somewhere at the border the train stopped, then continued, and somehow we arrived in Oldenburg."

Marte was ten at the onset of the war. On and off since 1940 she lived in evacuation camps. At the end of the war, she found herself in Oberschlesien. It was a time of the retreat of the German Army, "and with them . . . evacuated people . . . were returned, train after train. I was caught up in that, because we had to get out of Oberschlesien, through Czechoslovakia, partly on foot and then again with some sort of trains: freight trains, passenger trains, school groups, and old people—everyone mixed together. . . . We were emaciated, half-frozen and famished. In the end, nothing moved anymore. From then on . . . April 1945 . . . we walked through the Böhmerwald. . . . We older ones were assigned a younger child to watch and I got a ten-year-old girl . . . but such a wee one. And then, when we were in Pilsen a few days, the child died. Yes. She had diphtheria. . . . On and on [we walked] until we landed in a village called Neukirchen. And then I stayed there for years, in that village, together with some other sixteen year olds. What happened to all the others I don't know. A farmer took me in. I worked on the farm." Later, Marte found her way back to Berlin and found her mother. It was not the end of her trek. Back and forth across the border between East and West she went. She escaped to the West, away from the oppressive Russian domination. And then she returned—back to the East—to be with her kind mother.

Annette and her husband were living in the Russian-occupied zone of Germany after the war. They decided to leave. "My parents bid us goodbye and said they were too old. We should go West. We tried to swim across. It was soooo cold—it was May—that we returned home and dressed, and then went to hide ourselves inside a wagon loaded with hay. In the morning we heard gasping; it turned out to be a couple who were dying in the fields. Later we found a canoe in the bushes; we dragged it to the shore. It had but one paddle. We crossed and on the other side we mounted the bicycles we had taken with us and rode westward. In a village we asked whether there was a place we could stay . . . people were hospitable. . . . In the morning the woman said to me: 'I really am not allowed to tell you this, but your husband's boots are so nice, they can only be *SS*-boots.' In fact, they were riding boots . . . he had saved. . . . We left as fast as possible and rode on . . . with our bikes and the heavy bags with our worldly possessions hanging from them. . . . [We] raced down the field paths. Only fear kept us ensconced on top of our bikes. . . . [In a village] we worked on the farms. Americans interrogated us and released us again. . . . We left there when the news spread that the Americans were retreating. No one could understand that they gave a gift to the Russians of the land they had themselves conquered. . . . The fear! The fear was terrible."

Inge, born in 1920, was sent to Berlin to work. "In Berlin there was practically nothing. The food we got there was very sparse," she reported. She returned to Freiburg, her hometown, where "everything had been destroyed by bombs." By this time she "had a six-week old child and there was the constant worry to feed the baby. . . . I had to walk daily for an hour through the snow to get a liter of milk for my child. . . . We were actually starving and I had to steal. . . . I stole bread in a bakery. They knew me, [so] I went in at a time when I knew there would be no more bread in the front of the store . . . [went] in back where the baking was done, and there I stole the bread. Maybe they saw me . . . but people stole. I stole cabbage in the field. . . . I could have been reported, because I was not considerate of the welfare of the general population. . . . Once after a storm at night . . . I took the morning train [to a place] where there were apple orchards. We were allowed to pick up apples that had fallen, but when I came back to the train station with a rucksack full of apples, the police was there. They took away the apples and I was taken to the market square and had to stand there like traitor. . . . I was lucky. . . . I could have been sent to prison."

POSTTRAUMATIC STRESS

To be sure, there were those who had residual symptoms. One husband reported being awakened many a night for many years by his wife's shrieks at exactly two in the morning, the hour at which she had been raped by a Russian soldier. One woman recognized that her habits of laying out her clothes carefully before retiring each night and counting the steps of a stair-case in any house she visited had been useful when she suddenly needed to rush to the air-raid shelter in the dark of night. Now, in the absence of danger, these habits were unrealistic, anxiety-allaying compulsions.

Wilma said, "I can't stand the New Year's fire works, although basically I'm not fearful. When I hear that, I think, 'My God, that's how it was when the dive-bombers came.' One never loses the sense of those noises." For years, a number of interviewees continued to have nightmares; a few of them still do.

Heinz, the twelve-year-old guardian of little ones in the air-raid shelter, reported: "Even today I still dream about it often, the picture of the burning street, and of having to run, and the feeling of not being able to run."

Renate reported that, nowadays, when the planes break the sound barrier and the windows rattle, she is as if paralyzed. Slowly it's getting better.

Several women were aware of their tendencies to store and save foodstuffs, never to waste. Some were proud of their children, who had learned and practiced the many ways of making-do. Others were rather critical of their children who, having grown up in times of plenty, expected and granted themselves whatever they wished.

Inge, who had had to steal bread and pick fallen apples, later told her daughter, "You can do anything, but don't throw out bread. . . . I remem-ber the Americans after the war, how much they always threw away. That was painful."

Inge and two other women ascribed the origins of their physical symptoms to various sources. Inge thought the early onset and severity of her arthritis a result of the cold and hunger she suffered. The other woman said, "As soon as the sirens went off, I got diarrhea. After the war I had an ulcer. . . . You never get rid of something like that." A third one, an unmarried woman, complained of backaches. She intimated her problems were caused by the heavy physical work she had performed for years in her father's butcher establishment. Her physical and mental breakdown occurred toward the end of caring for her widowed, terminally ill mother.

The interviewer's impression was that, while Inge's problems probably had their roots in her unacknowledged dependency wishes underlying her manifest independence, the catalyst for her physical and psychological sufferings was the combination of wartime trauma, difficulties living and working under the supervision of a committed communist in East Germany, as well as her responsibilities caring for and then losing her ailing mother.

Despite these accounts, on the whole, this group of World War II children became accomplished adults. To questions about aftereffects of the war—such as those described by the shrieking wife, Inge, and several others—the great majority indicated nonverbally and verbally that such an idea had not crossed their minds. Yes, they had had rough times, but they had coped and now they were all right. What emerged from the interviews, overall, is that the traumatized German children coped, and most of them coped very well with the conditions of their lives.

It has been established that the nonclinical Holocaust population is far less symptomatic than the survivors who have sought psychotherapy; yet those who opt for psychotherapy tend to be more introspective.[8] Save one, the German child-survivors of the Nazi regime who volunteered to be interviewed did not undergo psychotherapy, and as a group they confirm the findings: Their plaintive reports were not at all introspective. Their accounts stressed the concrete, material events as they perceived them, and tended to emphasize their own and other people's actions—escape from bombs, flight from the Russians, rebuilding houses, contriving to finish school or to find work, and again and again, foraging for food.

"The absence of Posttraumatic Stress Disorder at long-term follow up, far from indicating that the trauma did not have a significant lasting impact, may rather imply that highly significant and idiosyncratic effects [may be found] . . . through exploration of the enduring patterns of adaption and their origins."[9] In this regard, I saw similarities between the Israeli pioneers and the post–World War II Germans: With their backs against the wall, in the face of danger and adversity, a pattern of intense striving for mastery and survival was activated in both groups. In a personal communication, Shamai Davidson noted that Holocaust survivors who devoted themselves vigorously to the building of Israel manifested few post-traumatic symptoms. Later, after retirement, after the cessation of daily distractions, and perhaps after some loss of strength and hope, many collapsed psychically and had to be hospitalized.

It is as if the German population, faced with virtually total destruction of their world, had to make gargantuan efforts to reconstruct their lives. Although rejecting Hitler's theories of racial superiority, during the interviews they spoke proudly of their achievements. Perhaps, unconsciously, they still saw themselves as *Übermenschen* (supermen), "invulnerables" who "test their strength even against overwhelming odds."[10] Like "invulnerables," the young Germans displayed an intense drive to master great risks, a high degree of confidence in achieving grand tasks, and an acceptance of the concomitant, necessary work, pain, punishment, and often loss. This is in stark contrast to fantasies of omnipotent grandiosity, characterized by a "hope to achieve great things with little work, pain, punishment or loss."[11] Nonetheless, not everyone who coped ultimately escaped the posttraumatic stress disorder. A 1964 study showed that the destruction of natural family ties is an important factor distinguishing symptomatic from symptom-free survivors.[12]

Barbara, who had to grow up overnight in December 1944, is an example of a young person whose family was broken up as a result of the war and who suffered late sequelae of her traumatic experiences. Bombed out and displaced, father and sister dead, she and her poor mother moved into the rather high-class paternal grandparents' home, where her father's sister also lived. No one wanted her because they wanted her hardworking mother's undivided attention and energy devoted to their business. Barbara thought a maternal aunt and her husband would have been a socially "appropriate family" for her, but the aunt had also perished and the uncle had remarried a "psychopathic," as she put it. Barbara was "practically thrown out of one family [and] the next day . . . sat at the other one's table." Barbara retreated into herself and matured quickly. She gritted her teeth and continued where she had left off. She could forget in school, but felt ten years older than the others. She didn't think her situation was unusual: Millions experienced similar conditions. She became a teacher and a volunteer, and was up to her ears in work. Did she become a workaholic to "forget" her wartime ordeals and family losses, as in school? Ultimately, she suffered a nervous breakdown. With the breakdown, the experiences of "that time" flooded her. Reading Mitscherlich, she concluded she hadn't mourned properly because prepubescent children reputedly are incapable of mourning.[13] For Barbara "the war has not ended. So long as there is someone who has lost a foot and hobbles and another who has inner injuries, the war isn't over. . . ."

COPING

It seems that adult mastery patterns are "laid down during overwhelming traumas encountered in the first twenty years of life," and they are at least partially based on an identification with a parent or parent surrogate.[14] To examine the intense urge for mastery as a response to traumatic experiences is not to dispute that, in some instances, prolonged stress, especially a threat to life, can result in a characterological regression, that is, to an "abandon-ment of structural and developmental achievements."[15] It had happened to Barbara. One can speculate that in her case the attempts at mastery were not integrated. Rather, she "forgot," had split off the pain associated with her wartime experiences and—fundamentally more important—the pain as-sociated with her family experiences.[16] The split laid the groundwork for the breakdown.

Current social or economic stress also can set in motion a revival of the traumatic situation, a sort of repetition compulsion. Anxiety may be de-fended against by splitting and projection, and these mechanisms may be utilized for governmental war propaganda. Thus, an individual's conscience can be undermined. This is apparently what occurred during the Nazi re-gime. The World War I generation—traumatized by the horrors of war, lack of food, and the postwar influenza epidemic—was at risk at the time of the subsequent monetary inflation and economic depression. Their experiences of absent fathers, anxious mothers, and the actual exigencies were reacti-vated. The threat of hunger mobilized primitive wishes for symbiosis and aroused a glorified father-image. Yearning for the father and the concomi-tant camouflaged homosexual wishes intensified the people's obsequiousness vis-à-vis the authority. German voters—including the 4 million, the 10 per-cent who reached voting age in 1930—confronting social disintegration and personal anxiety, gave themselves over to the promises and prejudices of a seemingly strong leader.[17] [18] And the psychic hollow left in the fatherless sons filled up with demons.[19]

On the other hand, adolescents who had endured hardships and had ob-served their parents cope with the trials of World War I and its sequelae later became the adult models for their children who learned to endure and cope with the disasters of World War II. Identifications with parental strengths "take on a preoedipal, oedipal, or later tenor, according to the epoch in which they were made," and depend on genetic endowment of ego capacities: intelligence, reflexes, and physical strength.[20] Insofar as chil-dren identify not only with their parents' coping behaviors, but also with their underlying values, these become the foundation for the children's su-perego. The superego is a "more conservative" carrier of cultural continuity than the ego in terms of "content and resistance to change."[21] The high value placed by Germans on industry, cleanliness, discipline, and toughness thus may be seen not only as a manifestation of an anal character organi-zation engendered by sadistic childrearing methods, but also as values that may become important guidelines to the striving for mastery in times of actual stress.

Mary reported coping at thirteen, when she helped out in an orphanage. The adult personnel had absconded toward the end of the war, and she was left to take charge of many little children, to take them for walks, for ex-ample. In autumn 1945, she returned to school. Solutions to the problems of a leaking roof, water on the floor, and lack of furnishings were planks to walk on and bringing one's own chair to sit on. She and her peers toughed it out. "We didn't suffer much," she said. "We were all basically glad to be alive, to be able to learn, and everything else didn't make a difference."

Willie could not believe what he heard and read after the end of the war. "We were, we were such brave Germans [clapped hands]. We said [clapped, laughed] we are brave. We are [clapped] committed to the righteous cause. For us the world collapsed . . . because we thought, *ja*, our position (*Sache*), our position is just. We hadn't heard anything about horrors. We only experienced the horrors here: the bombs, which . . . tore our families apart and shred people to pieces [claps]. The rest was far away." He had believed that the postwar magazines and newspaper reports were intentionally biased to influence the public and told himself, "Man-oh-man, our position is the just one; the other is evil. . . . It was a problem to sort things out." I asked what happened to him when he learned this confusing, unbelievable information. "*Tja*—[long pause]—you know, so much crashed in on us: the defeat, the lost war, then, eh, to see that one gets home; then to see that one—[long pause]—quiets the growling stomach. Then one had to make sure [claps] to fix up the apartment, at least halfway. . . . Continually one was running around: to get something to eat; continually we were on the go—[pause]—to find coal, eh, heating material—[pause]—one was only on the go . . . to fight for one's existence. One was so preoccupied with oneself, one couldn't think about things."

Willie was in Bayern at the end of the war, marching along with a group of teenagers in their workforce uniforms, trying to cope on their own, to survive without their leaders, and to find their way home from their assignments. The Americans thought they were young soldiers and shot at them. The boys ran and hid in the forest. Circuitously, they managed to reach a village where they spent the night at an inn. The next morning, when they heard the droning of tanks, they thought the Americans were coming to shoot them. When they cautiously looked out, they saw the German white flags hanging out and the *Amis* (Americans) coming through with their tanks, armed cupolas atop. The boys were surprised that the Americans didn't shoot them up, and then they thought, "Man, they're decent people after all . . . our arch-enemies. . . . We finally understood that, of course, they're people too."

Otto is a lively little man who grew up in a socialist family. He applied his ingenuity in every way to escape the Hitler-youth duties, though to be assigned an apprenticeship it was necessary to join. One day, he was accosted on the street by a chimney sweep, his face blackened by soot, who offered him ten marks to find a classmate who might be interested in learning the trade, because in 1940 they would need an apprentice. Everyone thought that a chimney sweep's work was too dirty, but the offer tickled Otto; he wanted the money badly. When they met again Otto said, "I have an apprentice, and I want the ten marks." "Where? Where is the apprentice?" the chimney sweep inquired. "I'm it!" he said, and stretched out his hand. "Got the ten marks. And so I began my apprenticeship." He went on to tell, "At that time nothing could be had without little chits: shoes, clothing, groceries, coal. One had to queue up. . . . I always took care of my family. I went to this dealer and that one and gathered stuff together . . . even after the war. . . . Through my work I was in strange houses every day and somewhere it always smelled of dinner: '*Hach*, it smells good,' I would say. 'Would you like a plate full?' '*Oh ja*,' so I always got my dinner or a piece of bread or something . . . and the farmers . . . gave me eggs as a tip . . . or onions, which were hard to get." It comes as no surprise that at the time of the interview Otto was an independent contractor, happy to be his own boss in the socialist German Democratic Republic (GDR, East Germany). And he was proud of his profession. "During the apprenticeship and vocational school the focus was really on the subject matter, not that political crap, not such shit they teach here."

Herta's complex story illustrates coping, identification with a parent, and the "abandonment of structural and developmental achievements," as postulated by Wangh.[22] In this case, a current social and economic stress set in motion a revival of the traumatic situation, a sort of repetition compulsion.

A local oral-historian had conducted one interview with Herta and asked me, the psychoanalyst, to come with him to the follow up. He was worried about Herta. I learned that Herta had led a rather protected, mildly privileged life in a coal mining town in the east. Her father had been a Nazi Party member, but to her knowledge was not actively engaged. He was needed in the coal industry, and therefore exempt from military service. (Though she did not know it, it was quite possible that he employed forced labor.) Toward the end of the war, her family had had to share quarters with a family evacuated from Berlin. The Berlin family had obtained a pistol and were making suicide plans. All they needed was someone to shoot. Her father, who in past times had been unable to help with the slaughter of a duck, now volunteered. The families were gathered in the hall, making plans. Herta cried, clung to her mother and said, "I don't want to. I don't want to. I'd rather hang myself." She, too, was afraid of the sight of blood. Her father said, "Allright, then you have to go to the attic. We are going to shoot ourselves . . . and whoever wants to leave, go. I am closing the door." Mother went with Herta, and grandmother joined them. As they climbed the stairs, they heard the shots. Everyone, including a five year old and a one-and-a-half year old perished.

Once upstairs, grandmother and mother had ropes around their necks, and mother fastened one around Herta's neck. Herta climbed up on the ladder. From there, she could look out of the skylight. She saw the sky and the clouds, and the April weather was beautiful. She thought, "Oh my God, I won't ever see this again." Then she didn't want to die. Again she began to cry and pleaded, "Perhaps it won't be so bad; let's wait; let's try." So the three women survived and left to live in grandmother's house in another town (Merseburg).

Mother, never before obliged to work for a living, now supported the family as a seamstress and encouraged Herta to study. Herta completed an academic high school program and the university curriculum in German literature and education. She married and, at age thirty-seven, had one daughter. Through a series of coincidences, she later became a painter and sculptress with her own studio.

At the time of the unification of East and West Germany in 1990, Herta felt like killing herself. "I am mourning," she declared. "If only I could cry. . . . If it were easy, I would kill myself [but] I'm too much of a coward." She was disappointed and disillusioned, hopeless and worried, like so many other East Germans: afraid she would be unemployed and struggling with a meager pension while prices rose to meet West German standards.

I suggested there might be a parallel between her suicidal thoughts during the demise of socialism in East Germany and her father's action at the time of the defeat of Nazism. She denied any identification with her father by alluding to their differences, and then she said, "For me, my father's death was not a suicide, rather the circumstances of the war . . . and the people were desperate. Now we have unusual times, but not war." But she added, "My surroundings are equally miserable and I don't have the strength" to put up a good front.

When I told her that she might be sad because she had three losses: her father, her fatherland, and now the GDR—and in addition had been disappointed even by her husband—she replied, "*Na ja*, I mean I'm a normal person, I'm not cracked. And now [when] I suddenly have doubts, you think that's normal?! I think it's stupid to howl and cry; and whether I have a good character or not, I'm full of hate. . . . Demonstrations, voting, nothing is important anymore—at least for the moment . . . but even if one takes one's life, it wouldn't change the problems."

Herta coped. She didn't give up. Over the years, she had made many friends whom she telephoned daily after this interview to talk about her depression. She credited them with seeing her through. She also had a little luck. When I saw her again in August 1991, she was happier. She was still able to afford her apartment and to maintain the studio for the time being. A West German banker on business in Berlin had seen her artwork on display at a café. He bought some paintings and arranged an exhibit of her work in West Germany.

A significant number of the interviewees had to cope with relocation and emigration; they had to leave their hometowns, which was uncommon and sad for Europeans of that generation (although it is not an unusual circumstance for Americans in the second half of the twentieth century). Relocation was forced upon many Germans by the population exchange, the flight from the Soviet army, the bombed-out houses, and the necessity of moving clear across the country for the sake of a lowly job. Some farmers or innkeepers offered shelter in return for work, but often the displaced individuals were neither welcomed nor helped, not even by relatives. For instance, when *Edith* asked to stay with a relative after her discharge from the hospital, she was refused with the excuse that Edith, still on crutches, would not be able to keep up should they have to run to a shelter or flee from the advancing troops.

Still, German citizens who had endured the air-raids, family disruptions, hunger, and relocation did have the benefit of certain advantages over other emigrant groups. They were not reviled and humiliated by their fellow burgers. They had the opportunity to remain in their German environment, live in their homeland, and speak their native tongue. German families had lost fathers or brothers on the battlefield, but generally individuals were not alone after their entire families had been deliberately wiped out, as was the case for so many Jewish survivors. To save their own lives, Germans did not have to cross oceans and to live among strangers.

Germans coped under more benign circumstances than those encountered by most Jewish emigrants. Nevertheless, today many still suffer homesickness and nostalgia. Speaking for many others, Rosa confessed that when she sees her sisters-in-law and her colleagues living in the communities and in the houses where they grew up, inside she shakes her head with envy and says, "Even in one's own country, one can be displaced!" (*"Man kann auch im eig'nen Land heimatlos sein!"*)

NOTES

1. Scott Turow, *The Laws of Our Fathers* (New York: Warner Books, 1996), 807.

2. These accounts are a very small part of the data collected during this author's research conducted in Germany between 1988 and 1992. See my articles: Charlotte Kahn, "Beleaguered Youth in a Collapsing Society," *The Journal of Psychohistory* 18, no. 1 (Summer 1990): 71–94; "Group Disjunction," *Psychoanalysis /Psychotherapy* 9, no. 2 (1991): 151–61; "Information Control and Distortion of Cognition: East Germans Review the Effects of Totalitarianism In Their Lives," *The Journal of Psychohistory* 19, no. 4 (Spring 1992): 409–20. "The Different Ways of Being a German," *The Journal of Psychohistory* 20, no. 4 (Spring 1993): 381–98; as well as note 4, below.

3. See chapter 12, this volume.

4. Daniel J. Goldhagen, *Hitler's Willing Executioners* (New York: Alfred A. Knopf, 1996), bases his conclusions on data pertinent to adults, not children, living in Nazi Germany.

5. In this work neither the selection of subjects nor the consistency of the interviews conform to strict standards of scientific research; however, during the interviews I did my level best not to introduce questions or comments that might convey my

own opinions. With two exceptions I also avoided making therapeutic interventions during the data collecting procedure. On a few occasions, there were postinterview moments that became more personal. For instance, as I was preparing to leave and as she lifted my coat from the hanger, one woman asked me about my background. I revealed that my parents had sent me out of Germany after *Kristallnacht* in 1938 and that I had come to the United States after a stay in Belgium and England. Then, when she found out my age—exactly the same as hers—she threw her arms around me and said, "To think we could have been classmates!"

6. Anna Freud, The *Ego and the Mechanisms of Defence* (1936; New York: International Universities Press, 1946), makes the point that some youngsters can take care of their juniors very well, even while they are childlike in other ways: dependent, submissive, and politically naive. They pander to their own, often unacknowledged, neediness by caring for others and generally taking charge of difficult situations, provided adults give guidance and maintain ultimate responsibility.

7. This man's interview material was riddled with evasions, generalizations, and rationalizations, casting doubt on the veracity of his statements.

8. Eva Fogelman, chapter 6, this volume.

9. Richard Honig et al., "Portraits of Survival: A Twenty-Year Follow-up of the Children of Buffalo Creek," in *The Psychoanalytic Study of the Child*, 53 vols. (New Haven, Conn.: Yale University Press, 1993), 48:327–55, quote cited on 351.

10. E. James Anthony and Bertram J. Cohler, eds., *The Invulnerable Child* (New York: Guilford Press, 1987).

11. Ibid.

12. W. von Baeyer, H. Häfner, and K. P. Kisker, *Psychiatrie der Verfolgten* (Psychiatry of the persecuted) (Berlin-Göttingen-Heidelberg: 1964); Paul Matussek, "Marriage and Family," in *Internment in Concentration Camps and Its Consequences* (1971; New York: Springer Verlag, 1975), 181–201.

13. Alexander Mitscherlich and Margarete Mitscherlich, *The Inability to Mourn* (New York: Grove, 1975).

14. Anthony and Cohler, *Invulnerable*, 315. Research was based on children who grew up traumatized by life with psychologically impaired parents. Nevertheless, the differentiation between omnipotent grandiosity and the establishment of a more realistic sense of mastery is useful for an understanding of a characterological ability to remain asymptomatic and competent in the face of adversity.

15. Martin Wangh, "Traumatization through Social Catastrophe," *International Journal of Psychoanalysis* 49 (1968): 319–31, quote cited on 320.

16. Matussek, "Marriage and Family."

17. Peter Loewenberg, "The Psychohistorical Origins of the Nazi Youth Cohort," *American Historical Review* 76, no. 5 (1971): 1457–1502.

18. Martin Wangh, "The Evocation of a Proxy," in *The Psychoanalytic Study of the Child*, 53 vols. (New York: International Universities Press, 1962), 17:451–69. Writes Wangh, "Through emotional surrender, object relationship is increased . . . a proxy serves to reinforce ego control, to maintain reality testing. . . ." Quote cited on 462.

19. Robert Bly, "Foreword," in Alexander Mitscherlich, *The Fatherless Society* (New York: Harcourt, 1993), xiv.

20. Edwin C. Peck, "The Traits of True Invulnerability and Posttraumatic Stress

in Psychoanalyzed Men of Action," in *The Invulnerable Child*, ed. E. James Anthony and Bertram Cohler (New York: The Guilford Press, 1987), 354.

21. Roy Schaefer, "The Loving and Beloved Superego," in *The Psychoanalytic Study of the Child*, 53 vols. (New York: International Universities Press, 1960), 15: 183.

22. Wangh, "Traumatization through Social Catastrophe."

17

My Contra-Program:
A Response to My Father

Gonda Scheffel-Baars

I was born in death, how can I learn to live?

I was born in December 1942 in the town of Rotterdam in Holland. I am my parents' second daughter. At the moment of my birth, my father was sitting at the foot of the bed, dressed in his Dutch National Socialist League (NSB) uniform. So I was literally born in the shadow of Nazism, the ideology of death.

This disgraceful, humiliating legacy plagued me for decades. I had to suffer exile and internment as well as ridicule. Yet, the psychological pain and impairment were considerably harder to bear. In that respect I am a child survivor: traumatized by war experiences and by discrimination—not because I am a Jew, but because I am the daughter of a Nazi collaborator.

This chapter is an account of my self-perception in relation to my father, and my struggle to gain sufficient self-esteem and confidence to overcome serious psychological and physical symptoms. I survived by means of my unconscious opposition to my father, my "contra-program." Later, as I grappled with the bad and the good, with hate and with love, a Protestant pastor, a Jewish psychologist, and a loyal, understanding mate helped me to embark on a normal course of life.

MY FATHER

Based on his interest in German philosophers like Schopenhauer and Nietzsche, my father had a positive inclination toward the National Socialist ideology as soon as it emerged in Germany. In the midst of war, in January 1942, he became a member of the NSB. He was then thirty years old and should have known that the Dutch saw his party as collaborative with the German enemies who had occupied the Netherlands since May 1940. Could he have foreseen the consequences of his choice? My mother did not agree with his decision to join the NSB, but in those days women were supposed to support their husbands' decisions and follow them blindly.[1]

I don't know why my father became a member or why he delayed doing so.[2] I wanted to find out, but he vehemently resisted discussions on the issue. For that reason, I started to study history. Perhaps the misery in his family of origin accounts to a large extent for his sympathies with the National Socialist Party, as it promised work and better social circumstances. My paternal grandfather was a farmhand, head of a family into which ten children were born, some of whom died in childhood. When there was no work, for instance in the winter season, he did not get any pay, and there was insufficient food and fuel for heating the house. There were only two chairs, so the children had to stand around the table during meals. They never ate meat, sometimes one or two eggs, and at Christmas, the church gave oranges as presents. My father was the second son, the only strong child in the family, of good health and a more than moderate intelligence. After primary school, he went to work to earn money for the family, continuing his studies at a technical school in the evening. When my father was fifteen years old, my grandfather died and my father assumed responsibility for the family. Ultimately, he became director of the most important Dutch shipbuilding company in Brazil.

When he finished his studies in 1936, however, he could not find a job because of the lingering effects of the Great Depression of 1929. This was a deep disappointment: Now he had to return to a life of poverty.

Another reason that may have prompted him to become a NSB party member can be found in the anticommunist attitude of the orthodox Protestant population to which he belonged. To fight communism was almost a religious duty; fighting communism meant resisting atheism. This might explain why, in January 1942, father asked to be sent to the eastern front. His request was refused because of his imperfect eyesight. Nor was he allowed to join the "Storm Troopers" (SS) or other semimilitary groups.

On the basis of testimony given by an uncle, who was present at the court when my father's case was read, I know that my father was sentenced for his membership in the Party and also for some negative statements about Queen Wilhelmina, who had fled to London. My uncle, a staunch Protestant, told my mother the truth, I am sure. So I believe my father did not kill or betray anyone. Still, he is responsible for his choice to support a criminal Nazi system, responsible for the consequences of this choice, and responsible for the effects on the victims of this system, the Dutch people, and our family. He always denied his guilt, claiming that because the Party was not declared to be an illegal organization until 1945, members cannot be accused retrospectively. But he overlooked the moral aspect of this "legal" membership.

Like so many other collaborators' children, I had loaded my father's guilt on my own neck. I always felt that such guilt should not be suppressed. It had to be confessed, and, whereas my father did not, I did so in his place. In 1975, I wrote a letter to the *Jerusalem Post* and confessed my father's guilt. Samuel Cohen from Nahariya, Israel, answered me—in French! Nine years later I visited him during my first stay in Israel.[3] In his letter he stressed that I had the right to love my father for the mere fact of his being my father, notwithstanding his guilt. From that time on, I could start trying to unburden myself. It was a difficult job.

MY MOTHER

My mother was the fifth child in her family; another five were born after her. My grandfather had been a radical socialist in his twenties. He was also a vehement opponent of the use of alcohol or tobacco. In the course of his career, he became the director of a bank catering to workers in the needle trades and of middle-class enterprises. He was an authoritarian person. Although the family was fairly wealthy and had two housemaids, all the daughters were engaged in the housekeeping without pay; they were treated more or less like slaves. They were brought up in obedience while the sons had far more freedom. The family belonged to a little Protestant church, the Seventh Day Adventists, in which people observed several traditions of Jewish origin, such as the celebration of the Sabbath on Saturday instead of on Sunday.

WARTIME

During the last period of the war, my mother, my older sister, and I were in a refugee camp in Germany. As the Allies advanced, the NSB leaders had advised women and children to seek safety in the Third Reich, so in early September 1944, when I was one-and-a-half years old, we left Holland. Sixty-five thousand Dutch women and children relocated in the north of Germany at the time. The local people were rather reluctant to accept us, to give us shelter and food.

The only word I spoke while in Germany was "no." It was my own expression of resistance against everything that happened. I became an "impossible" child. In retrospect I feel this attitude helped me to survive. In Germany I suffered from dysentery and was sent to a hospital. Believing I would have a better chance to recover there, my mother did not oppose the move. For me, however, it was a traumatic experience. I did not understand why my mother had abandoned me. A child cannot understand that it is "for her own good" that she has to stay all alone in a hospital in a strange country where people speak another language. Recently I have come to realize that my panic during present misunderstandings and miscommuni-

cations can be traced to the distress and agony suffered by the little girl in
that foreign hospital.

In February 1945 we returned to the Netherlands, but we could not
return to Rotterdam, for the western part of the Netherlands was still isolated due to a strike of railway employees, ordered by the London-based
Dutch government in exile. In the north of Holland, people in villages were
forced to open their houses to the women and children who came back
from their evacuation. The atmosphere in the house to which we were assigned was rather good. In contrast, on Holland's liberation day, the women
and children of the collaborators were summoned to a factory that had been
set up as an internment camp, and the villagers alongside the road shouted,
insulted us, and spat at us. Although we were not guilty, they unloaded on
us all the hatred they had accumulated during five years of war. My own
people rejected me and cut me off. They reduced me to a mere object. Had
they truly seen me, they would have seen an innocent child and would have
prevented me from being imprisoned. This was my "liberation day." Now
I can understand their attitude: It was difficult for them to distinguish between the collaborators and their innocent wives and children. It took a
long time for some people in the Netherlands to learn to make the distinc-
tion, and even nowadays, the older generation continues to view us, the
guiltless children, as collaborators.

In the Dutch internment camp, I again fell ill. I managed to survive,
thanks to an aunt who visited the camp and took my sister and me away.
For a long time I thought that my first memory was of sitting among the
strawberries in my uncle and aunt's garden, of the sun's warmth on my skin,
birds in the sky, of this calm and harmony after my recovery. In short, I
remembered paradise. Consciously, I did not remember the chaos of the
war, the flight, or the refugee camp in Germany; yet I was aware of a tension
somewhere in my body and in my mind. Recently my mother confirmed a
repetitive picture in my mind: the latrine in the camp, open and dirty with
an awful filth, and my being terribly afraid that I would tumble down into
the shit. The woman to whose house we had been assigned before being
sent to the Dutch camp helped by bringing a chamber pot for me, and so
delivered me from this horror.

Years later, when I interviewed some people who had been in institutional
homes set up for NSB children for my M.A. essay, they told me that the
nurses had failed to call for medical help when children were ill and that
some had even said, "Let them die, then we have one problem less." Weak
and thin, I had been such a "problem." It is bitter to acknowledge that,
although the Nazis were murderers of millions, the Germans in fact had
allowed me to recover in a hospital, whereas my own people, who saw themselves as the "good ones," did not take care of me.

My father, who had neither accompanied us to Germany nor been with us at liberation day, the day we were arrested, went into hiding. He showed up some weeks after our arrest to visit my mother in the detention camp, while my sister and I were at my aunt's house. After that visit, the son of the family that had housed us denounced my father. He was arrested and convicted of being a traitor supporting the German occupiers. My mother, on the other hand, was released after fourteen weeks, when an initial inquiry revealed that she had not been a Party member. She joined my sister and me, and after some weeks in my paternal grandmother's crowded little house, we went to my mother's parents. They allowed us to live in their large and luxurious home. My grandparents and an aunt tolerated but did not really welcome us; yet their house became a safe haven to me. It was my shelter against a threatening world.

After the War

When my sister went to kindergarten, the principal introduced her to the teacher with disdain and hatred: "This is an NSB child." My mother was upset, but what could she do? This is how many NSB children were treated, and in fact, my sister and I were spared much of the humiliation and teasing others had to endure. Without knowing why, we were wary. We suspected there was something dramatic and dangerous in our lives that had to be kept secret. But what? Once I hummed a song I must have remembered my father singing. He became furious! It was a forbidden song, and he feared that I would sing it at school or at the neighbors'.

My father came home from his internment in 1948. I was five years old. He was a complete stranger to me, although I had visited him several times in the detention camp. I remember those trips and the visits, but not my father. As soon as he was home, he took upon himself the task of being the head of the family. He intervened during the very first meal we were eating together because I was spilling the food. I watched him with disdain, thinking, "Who are you to tell me how to eat? If anybody has to tell me, it is my mother." Soon I realized that from now on, it was he who held the power. I submitted, but I never accepted it. I became afraid of the authoritarian man and never managed to overcome the emotional barrier in our relationship erected by the confrontation on that first day. I have always felt very guilty about this. He rebuked me again and again, although at the beginning he had sweet names for me and played with my sister and me. Now I feel, though, that it is the responsibility of adults—even ones as frustrated as my father was after his detention—to establish a good relationship with a child, not that of a five-year-old child paralyzed by fear.

At school, at the age of eight, I heard about the war. The teacher spoke about the traitors—who were depicted as the "rotters," the evil ones—and he told us about the resistance fighters—the good ones. By then, I understood what our secret was and why the "good" people had rejected us. I knew my father was such a "rotter." I had already become accustomed to keeping quiet and staying in the background; from then on, I consciously remained silent. We isolated ourselves in order to prevent people from rejecting us once more. In those days, the population was considered to have been "good," excepting the 5 percent who had been collaborators. Only in the 1960s and 1970s did people start to realize that 90 percent had been bystanders. Still, the myth of the "good" Dutch people is deeply rooted.

ENDURING MY AUTHORITARIAN FATHER

I had fewer conflicts about my poor relationship with my stern father than did those NSB children of warm and helpful fathers. I saw only his bad side, and later had to work at seeing and accepting his positive points. In the long run, I got a more realistic picture of him and came to learn to love him.

I do have some good memories of my father. When he was in the internment camp, he wrote letters to my sister and me about fairy tales of elves and pixies and of animals in the forest helping each other in disastrous and difficult times. After his detention, he told us stories while we lay at his side, after my mother had left the bed to prepare breakfast. This became a Sunday morning ritual. We also played together on Sundays and, despite my angry feelings toward him, that was nice.

Unfortunately, the bad memories are more numerous and more vivid. Once, when my sister or I had forgotten to put new toilet paper in the basket after we had used the last pieces, he reacted furiously and shouted, "You did this in order to tease me," showing how frustrated he was.

Father was a harsh taskmaster. When I had made a mistake or had been disobedient, he forced me to copy the longest poem in a book he had. When, as an act of resistance against his authoritarian behavior, I sometimes slammed the door behind my back, I was forced to open and to shut the door quietly ten times. Usually I could not resist the impulse to shut the door more loudly on the tenth time; then I was forced to perform the whole ceremony again. This punishment was effective because during the ensuing months I was obedient. When I had taken off my shoes without untying the laces, I had to put the laces in and take them out, ten times. And, of course, we also learned this lesson.

At one time, my mother was embroidering with wool. She had made two braids of the wool. I took them and hung them around my ears. As I had very thin hair, I felt like a princess with these beautiful brown tresses, and walked around the room, enacting a fairy tale in which I had the principal role. My father became irritated and urged me to put down the tresses. When he was absorbed in his reading, I took them and went upstairs to my room to continue the play. Suddenly he was there, pulled them off, and shouted, "I had forbidden you to have them on your ears." *Befehl ist Befehl!*

(A command is a command!) Here he was a real Nazi, not understanding that my playing fairy tales at the age of eight was a flight from the threatening world. He said I was too old for such childish things. He did not allow me to be just what I was: a child.

The only time my father came close to confessing guilt was one afternoon when my pen made a big blot of ink in the dictionary. I was scared because this was an expensive book, and although my father allowed my sister and me to have a good education, he always stressed the fact that he had to work very hard because the tuition was high. I feared his anger, and during that whole afternoon I was scared. How to face his fury? Strangely enough, just before he came home, I had put the whole thing out of my mind. But fate was playing against me: My father wanted to check a word in the dictionary. Suddenly I remembered my "crime," jumped to my feet, and wanted to tell him before he saw the damage in the book, but he had already found it and asked who was the perpetrator. When I told him, he became furious and tore the page from the book. That was too much for me, and I ran to my bedroom and wept. My mother came and urged me to stop weeping and come downstairs in order to apologize. I refused this half-hearted intervention. I wept and wept and could not stop anymore. After a long time, my father came to my room. I don't remember whether he said anything. In any case, I felt his coming as an expression of remorse on his part. Then I could stop crying. He wrote a letter to my teachers saying that I had not been able to do my homework.

After we left the shelter of my grandparents' house, I found a second hold on life at school. I was intelligent and always the best pupil in my class. My grades were better than those of my sister, who was much taller and stronger than I and was, moreover, my father's darling. This became my instrument to compete with her. Although my need to be the best one was neurotic, I had no problems reaching the highest academic level. I excelled in almost all subjects and performed quite well even in sports. I hoped thereby to gain the attention and perhaps the love of my father; I hoped he would praise me and notice my existence. Though he could not ignore my success and boasted about them to his colleagues, the praise I got was small: "Of course children do their best."

Yet, in one area I was far from the best. In my father's eyes I was the shame of the family. When I was twelve, I had to sleep in a bed of plaster in order to correct some problems with my back. When I came home from the clinic, my father forced me to lie down in that bed and to show it to the whole family. I felt terribly embarrassed in my underwear, but he had no mercy. In retrospect, I felt as if I was in a coffin, with an insensitive family standing around me. The Nazi ideology had strongly influenced my father's opinions to the extent that before his marriage he had gone with my mother to a physician to check for genetic problems. (I always wondered whether he would have sent my mother away had any genetic problems been revealed.) Father enjoyed good health and took it for granted, disdaining all those who were weak. He had always blamed people with handicapped children, advocating that the government forbid people with hereditary diseases to have offspring. Now I was a handicapped child and a shame for the family! Again I felt that I should not have been there, so that there would be "one problem less."

LEAVING HOME AND FINDING A MATE

I left the academic high school at sixteen to study French at a vocational high school. I left because I was too young, too childish, and because of an incident with a professor. When my professor—I still don't know why—asked me, who had not yet even kissed a boy, whether I was pregnant, I became so upset I could no longer concentrate on my work. My grades plummeted. Of course, I did not dare tell my parents, for fear of my father's anger. Not succeeding in school was a severe blow to me; my only hold on life broke. Again my father added fuel to the fire, declaring, "Yes, you are no longer that clever girl." I developed an eating disorder, close to anorexia, and my parents became afraid. They sent me to a psychiatrist, who advised me to leave my parents' house and to go to live in town. Sitting in front of his desk I thought, "Not I, but my father should be sitting here."

I went to The Hague, found a job in an office, and felt terribly alone. I feared I would commit suicide. However, I found my creative talents were still intact. So I decided to enroll in the teacher-training college to become a primary-school mistress, my childhood dream; once again school helped me to regain some self-confidence. I made friends and even fell in love. It was there that I met my future husband. He was patient when listening to me and inventive in curing me of my eating problems.

On our second date, I told him about my father's past. I did not want to take the risk of falling in love only to be rejected when the truth came out. Many collaborators' children had had such bad experiences, but my future husband reacted well. He said, "I want you, not your father. We have nothing to do with him." Had we known how deeply I had been influenced by my father's decisions and the resulting discrimination, I am not sure we would have had the courage to marry. But even then it was clear that I did not want to have children of my own, although, like my husband, I was fond of children. I did not want to continue the chain of evil, harm, and trouble.

Getting Help

When my father decided to go to Brazil in 1967 to represent the shipyard where he was employed, my mother did not object. I protested because I was concerned about my seventeen-year-old brother, who also developed problems concentrating on his studies after my father's past was revealed. However, my father was not swayed by my objections, and my parents departed in the spring of 1968.[4] I felt so upset that I contacted a pastor. He gave me a new perspective. "Come along and we will discuss things," he said. "I don't guarantee a solution, but I am ready to go down into the pit together with you. If we lose our way, we will be together." TOGETHER! Never had an adult said such a wonderful word to me. During our continued contact it became clear that the source of my problems was in my father's past. Fourteen years later, this pastor initiated our self-help group *Herkenning* (Recognition) and asked me to join the leadership.

At eighteen, I became a church member. In my faith, I found a new hold on life. Becoming a church member was most important, as I see it now. On the basis of my faith, I decided that if I could conceive, I should no longer resist having children. If I believed in "the new heaven and the new earth," the messianic era, I had to believe that there was a future for me and my children. This was a firm step forward from despair to hope! I thought it silly that a psychiatrist who supervised the German self-help groups (in which I participated for four years) interpreted this by saying, "So you, too, dedicated your children to a Führer [meaning, to God]." Her jargon may be appropriate to her profession, but could she not look beyond the religious terms I used and see them as an expression of my choice for life?

Two sons were born to us. The pregnancies were difficult, the deliveries easy. My second son was deathly ill when he was just seven weeks old, and I suffered from postpartum depression. I feared I should kill my children in a moment of despair. But the medicines calmed me, and thanks to God, apart from some unfair behavior toward my children, I never did attack them.

When we were moving to another house, not too far away, I learned how not-remembered events play a role. My second son, then one-and-a-half years old, was deeply upset. He missed his house, and although he had his own bed, his toys, his parents, and his beloved brother around, he felt unhappy, bumped his head against the wall, and medication was necessary to calm him. Then I realized how significant these experiences are and remembered my having been in Germany, in the refugee camp, and in Holland in the internment camp, at about the same age as my little son at the time of the move. If a prepared-for move could cause such a sense of uprootedness in a child, what had happened to me? I was afraid and lacked the courage and energy to explore this question. One year later, I could no longer escape. I had to start my working-through.

My mother had contacted a pastor after listening to his radio program. The pastor had spoken first about the love of God and then praised a book that attacked collaborators. Suddenly my mother became very angry, overcame her fears, and phoned him. She asked him when this hatred would stop because, again and again, the innocent wives and children of collaborators were met with hatred. At first, he did not want to listen to her because he had been in a concentration camp, but my mother persisted and told him about her own experiences in the camps. He heard her and then told her that she had opened his eyes to an issue he had never wanted to face. Still trembling, my mother phoned first my sister, and then called me to get my reaction. My sister was afraid; she did not want our names mentioned. My first reaction, inside my heart was: Oh no, not now that there is some calm in my life, don't pull me into your problems. Yet, this was the decisive moment! I realized, in 1974, in a free country, we were still as afraid as if it were wartime or as if we were living in a totalitarian state. I wanted to leave my prison, my ghetto of silence. I backed my mother, told her she did a good thing, and then wrote a long letter to this pastor to tell him my side of the story. I ended the letter by telling him, "You can betray us, as did other pastors whom my mother contacted, by neglecting their professional vow to keep silence; or you can prove you are worthy of the confidence we gave you." I went to the post office, but made several rounds before I had the courage to put the letter in the mailbox. Like my husband, the radio pastor reacted well. We had a good contact for several months. It made a deep impression on me that not all people would reject me once they knew of my father's past. I found that, having had the courage to break the silence and having received a good response from the pastor, I had the courage to talk with others as well. After each such conversation, I felt tired and disoriented, but also relieved.

IN SEARCH OF MY FATHER

Very soon after the start of my working-through, I realized I hated my father because of what he had inflicted on us. Recognizing this hatred was a big step forward. The next step was asking myself if there was something more. I continued to seek a better understanding of my relationship with my father, and nowadays I feel that the seeking is already one aspect of love. I could accept my father as soon as I was able to distinguish between the criminal Nazi system (or any totalitarian system) and the human beings who adhered to it. I learned to allow for the social, economic, and ideological contexts in which people made their decisions. In 1975 I wrote this in a letter to my father, but lacked the courage to give it to him. My fear of his rejecting me once more was so intense that I kept the letter. One year later, he died suddenly. Although I had not told him, I felt relieved to have accepted him.

It was fourteen years later, in the course of a therapy-by-letter with an Israeli psychologist friend, that I came to feel closer to my father. First, I had to work through the bad memories. On the way to my teaching job—during the half-hour trip through the quiet polders (reclaimed lowlands in

Holland), where there was hardly any traffic and I did not risk an accident—
I imagined one of the emotional scenes and tried to conjure up the feelings
of the past. Then I started to cry, to shout, to feel helpless, or angry. I
replayed such scenes until I could face them without overwhelming feelings.
Good memories came back afterward. When my friend suggested to me that
my father might have had a sexual relationship with another woman, I described the religious context in which he was raised and explained that such
a relationship would have been the very last thing my father would have
engaged in. I told him how my father's life had been influenced by my
grandmother's rape by her boss, the town's respected baker, resulting in an
out-of-wedlock child two years before she found a man willing to marry her;
and how, at the age of fifteen, when his father died, he defended his flir-
tatious sisters' honor, trying to prevent them from flirting and going out,
and prevailing on his mother to punish them when they returned later than
the arranged time. Then it suddenly became clear that these events had
influenced me as well. Although I knew about the transfer of traumas of
war and oppression, by the very fact of their having been silenced by the
survivor-parents, I had not realized that this can be true for all kinds of
traumas, including sexual scandals and related taboo family themes.

As I always felt like an orphan in my parental home, like a child fallen
from heaven into just anyone's house, I had not thought beyond myself. I
had not considered my parents' life and that of my grandparents. Suddenly
I felt my family roots; I cried because of my grandmother's fate, cried for
my father, and cried for myself. Some weeks later, my psychologist friend
suggested that the warm feelings I was conveying to him actually belonged
to my father. "There is the angry little girl that does not want to give her
father her love." Despite my initial feeling that this analysis was wrong, it
ultimately gave me the key! As my father had rejected the love I had offered
him and as I still wanted emotional contact with him, the only thing to do
was to offer him this love one more time. Although he had been dead for
many years, I felt scared when I sat down at the table to write him a letter.
It was difficult not to beat about the bush. But as soon as I had written
down how abandoned I had felt each time my father rebuked me, I felt
relief. An incredible calm filled me. I felt he had accepted my love, accepted
me. Then I had the courage to ask him to give me his blessing. He did. Of
course, this happened only in my mind, in my heart. I left my fears behind
and saw my love as more important than his rejection. The strength of this
love is mine; nobody can snatch it away. My father ceased being a negative
influence in my life. Though he never became a positive influence, my feelings are now in harmony and, for me, he rests in peace.

The "Contra-Program"

Like many other collaborators' and Nazi children, unconsciously—but in retrospect very clearly—I developed a "contra-program" to that of my father.

In contrast to my father, the traitor, I became a Girl Scout and promised to serve God and my country. While my father was charged with having slandered the Queen, I, as a Girl Scout, was received in audience by her daughter, Queen Juliana.

My father hated Jews, although he might never have met one. He supported a system that aimed at the annihilation of the Jewish people. On the other hand, I found my hold on life in my faith and discovered during my studies of history that the roots of Christianity lay in Judaism. I studied Hebrew and Jewish history, and discovered in Judaism the religious, ethical, and cultural material for the building of my house of life.

My father, as an adherent of the Nazi doctrine of eugenics, disapproved of and discriminated against handicapped people. I participated in groups for handicapped Girl Scouts; I was inspired by their acceptance of their handicaps. My father despised black and colored people, whereas I developed a close relationship with some Moluccan women who, forced to come to Holland when expelled from Indonesia (the former Netherlands East Indies) in 1950, had been virtually abandoned by our government.

In my life, however, I have more than a contra-program. In some ways, I followed in my father's footsteps. He had an analytic mind, and I inherited this gift. He liked to read and to write, and so do I. I am interested in questions of theology, philosophy, history—in the same way my father took an interest in them.

As a boy, my father studied in the evening because he had to work during the day, and now I am a teacher in a school where working adults are given a second chance. With my work in this school I honor my father and all those who were granted too few opportunities.

My father had a negative attitude toward women, which also infected me. I experienced the women of my childhood and youth as rather vulnerable and dependent and not very inspiring. I did not want to be like them. My mother never held a job, did not have money of her own, and was dependent. In my marriage, I had some emancipation clashes with my husband, but, in the end, it was he who stimulated me to continue my studies at the university. During my course of study, I met several inspiring women who influenced me in a positive way. So I found an outlet in my intellectual development, although I did not neglect my emotional development. Thus, I also developed a contra-program to that of my mother.

A contra-program is born out of unconscious resistance to the parents and can remain in this stage of rebellion. It can also emancipate one and then become a program in its own rights. For example, my interest in Judaism was born out of feelings of guilt toward the Jewish people. Later, as I learned the wealth of its concepts, I involved myself in the study of Judaism for its inherent qualities. During my first trip to Israel, an old rabbi provided a wonderful answer when one of our group asked him about "the sins of the fathers which are visited by God upon the third and fourth generations." He reproached the young theologian who had asked the question for having stressed but one part of the text and neglected the second, more important part, which stated (said the rabbi) "God gives mercy and grace to thousands of them who love Him and follow His commandments." Moreover, he explained that the second generation, though influenced by the wrong choices of the parents, nevertheless has its own opportunity and responsibility to return to virtuous ways. And if the children do so, they receive a reward: grace for the offspring, extending even beyond the third and fourth generations. Although I could not grasp the full significance of his answer at that moment, now, years later, I feel that by my own moral decisions, I can repair some of the damage caused by my parents and my ancestors. It was my task to pursue this course, and although it has not been an easy path, I feel I have been loyal to my calling.

BETRAYAL AND SHAME; REPENTANCE AND CHANGE

During and immediately after the war, the Dutch members of the NSB, the SS, the *Waffen-SS*, and other Nazi organizations were seen by the Dutch people as traitors because they supported and cooperated with the German occupiers. Inside the Party, however, there were variant factions: one rigid strain that followed the codes of the Third Reich in detail, and the other, a nationalistic group that did not support the "Great German" concept. For that reason, a simplistic notion of traitor is not applicable. Until now, there has been very little research concerning the motives of those who became NSB members. In this connection, a prominent Dutch historian of World War II voiced his impressions at a meeting of our self-help organization for children of collaborators. It was his opinion that the majority of NSB members never aimed at the betrayal of their native country; rather, they were blind to the negative consequences of Nazism and driven by economic, social, opportunistic, and ideological motives. They were anticommunistic and sometimes had antisemitic ideas, nurtured by the church. Interviews with fifty-two prominent collaborators, exploring possible psychological preconditions to joining the Party, also revealed that social and economic conditions were more likely to be decisive than psychological factors.[5]

Soon after the liberation from the Nazi occupation, the accusation could be heard occasionally that the NSB members had been active in the deportation of Jews. For example, one five year old was welcomed to the children's home (similar to, but not the same as an orphanage) with, "Your parents killed the Jews; it would have been better if they had sent you, too, to the gas chambers." Such accusations became more prevalent in the sixties and the seventies, when public attention at last turned to the question of genocide. Nowadays, the Jews find the courage to state openly that they were met with antisemitism even after the war. They feel abandoned by the Dutch people as a whole. And they know that the concept of the "good" Dutch people is a myth.

The television movie *Holocaust* made people aware of what had happened. Both during and after the war, the Dutch people had made rigid distinctions between the right and the wrong, overlooking the fact that only 5 percent of the Dutch population had been in the resistance and 90 percent were bystanders. This rigid division still plays an important role in Dutch society. However, as the citizens realize their sense of helplessness vis-à-vis the enemies; as they recognize their unawareness at the time when Jews had to live in a quasi-apartheid society; as they acknowledge their religious and political prejudices; and as they confront their reluctance, during that era, to help Jews and other refugees, the people's shame and guilt may give rise to the need to seek a scapegoat. The collaborators, as well as their wives and children, are easily identified scapegoats.

Two occurrences may show how little the tendency to appoint and to blame a scapegoat has been worked through. Fifteen years ago, it was revealed that the leader of the Christian Democratic Party had been a member of the *Waffen-SS*. His political party had known of his more or less forced participation in the Nazi organization at the age of twenty, and had accepted his confession of guilt and repentance. The Dutch people, however, asked for his resignation. Despite his positive attitude toward Israel, his social-work activities, and his support of financial organizations for the benefit of Jews, he remains suspect to most of the Dutch. Neither his detention nor his confession of guilt could lift the ban. In fact, he was sentenced to life imprisonment.

A few years ago, twenty-five Jewish women asked the Yad Vashem to decorate Alfons Zundler with a Medal of Righteousness. Zundler was an *SS* man who had helped them to escape from *De Hollandsche Schouwburg*, a Dutch theater where Jews had been concentrated before deportation. Immediately after the publication of the proposal in the *NIW (New Israelite Weekly*, a newspaper), a committee was formed, protesting against this demand for an award. They argued that Zundler had required alcohol and sex for his services, and supported their position with testimonies from some former German enemies, who claimed Zundler had been convicted of *Rassenschande* (literally, disgracing the race; a Nazi term for sexual relations with a nonaryan). The Jewish women, in turn, registered complaints, objecting to the priority given to the German testimony at the expense of their own.[6]

I understand that in 1945 people were still suffering the shock of the war and, therefore, needed a structure that could help them make a new start. The good-bad, right-wrong schema was such a structure. Time was not yet ripe for most of the Dutch to have a more differentiated opinion. Even today, this black-white schema allows them to avoid facing difficult questions, and many do not see the need for a change of mind. This need for a split appears to me to be deeper among the Dutch than in some other western European peoples. Perhaps we can discern here the remaining influence of the Dutch roots in Calvinism. According to one Calvinist concept, a perpetrator is not seen as someone who made a mistake, or made the wrong decision, or did a bad thing. No. *He* is bad, evil incarnate. The other concept is that of predestination: God has decided that some people will be saved and others will perish. Man's own role is of little or no importance in the divine schema. Right is right and wrong is wrong. Although few people adhere to Calvinist orthodoxy, Dutch public opinion in fact reflects the old doctrines, the belief that a perpetrator can never evolve to a higher moral level.

Thus, to split the bad from the good is an attempt to deny our own potentiality for evil by projecting it onto a scapegoat. Denial leaves us helpless to face our evil. It serves our need to see Nazis as monsters, while avoiding the troubling reality that very normal people can turn into "devils." We remain helpless in the face of evil if we continue to avoid the question of destructiveness in all humankind—in ourselves, as well as in the actual perpetrators.

Furthermore, we deceive ourselves as long as we deny the possibility of change. As long as we do not wholeheartedly recognize people's ability to repent and change, we block our own working-through and that of the perpetrators.

The children of Nazis and collaborators had to face and explore the evil in all of us. We must also accept the potentiality of, and responsibility for, remorse and altruism.

EPILOGUE

After completing this text, and on the occasion of the commemoration of the Liberation of the Netherlands from the Nazis, I sent a letter to Her Majesty, Queen Beatrix, alerting her to the continuing difficulties experienced by the children of Dutch collaborators and the self-help activities designed to help us work out and perhaps rid ourselves of the burdens of our heritage. Referring to the Belgian King Albert's appeal to his people—finally, after fifty years, to end the divisive strife between the "rights" and the "wrongs" (the collaborators)—I asked her "to launch a similar appeal to our people [for the sake of] the collaborators' children."[7]

On Christmas 1994, and again addressing the Israeli Knesset in Spring 1995, the queen delivered a speech introducing a new, conciliatory view, a breakthrough: No longer do the Dutch people dare tease and scapegoat the children of collaborators—not even their parents.[8]

NOTES

1. The NSB was legally organized in 1931, and although in 1934 the Dutch government forbade their functionaries to become members, the Party was never outlawed in the Netherlands. Indeed, one-and-a-half years after the German occupation, all other political activities were forbidden, and the NSB became the only recognized and authorized party.

2. I can speculate that my father joined after the Dutch NSB leader had visited Hitler and pledged loyalty to him in December 1941, and the Party accepted new members. It is also possible that my father wanted to participate in the war against the communists, which at that time still promised victory for the Germans.

3. Samuel Cohen's letter of April 25, 1975, translated by the author, reads as follows:

Dear Madam,
We read your letter in the paper of Israel with much emotion. Thank you for your good wishes and for all your prayers. As to us, my family and I, we send you sincere wishes, hoping you will recover soon and we pray to God with all our heart for your convalescence. Thank you for your sincere friendship; we love all our brothers belonging to whatever religion. . . .
P.S. Excuse me: as I could be your father (I have a daughter of your age), I take the liberty to say to you: don't judge your parents, respect their memories, it is only up to God to judge us. I embrace you with love. P.S. If you ever have the opportunity to visit Israel, I would like to have you as a guest in my family. S. Cohen.

At the beginning of my visit he seemed to be testing me, my participation in the study trip exploring the relationship between the Jewish and Christian religions. Our three-hour encounter ended with the reading of some Yom Kippur prayers.

4. My parents returned to the Netherlands in the autumn of 1969, Brazil having confiscated the shipyard as part of the nationalization process.

5. Interviews were conducted by the psychiatrist Dr. T. Hoffmann, one of the founders of the self-help organization *Herkenning*.

6. Hennie Beek-Gobitz and Carla Kaplan-Gobitz, "Zündler 15," *Niew Israelitisch Weekblad* (New Israelite Weekly) November 26, 1993; Suzanne Glass, "Will Honoring *SS* Guard Dishonor Yad Vashem?" *Jerusalem Post International Edition* (June 4, 1994), 12.

7. Gonda Scheffel-Baars, letter dated October 10, 1994. Mine was not the only letter.

8. Konigin Beatrix, *De Telegraaf* Amsterdam, December 27, 1994, T4.

Afterword

Charlotte Kahn

We cannot—we will not—succumb to the dark impulses that lurk in the
far regions of the soul, everywhere. We shall overcome them, and we
shall replace them. . . . [1]

—President William Clinton

The "dark impulses that lurk in the far regions of the soul" are difficult to
contain and to control. Hostile aggression is impossible to eradicate and
only the greatest vigilance and empathy will replace prejudice, xenophobia,
and contempt with humane concern. Clearly threat, fear, humiliation, competition, and primordial strivings for survival all arouse hostility in the human animal. The accounts in this anthology demonstrate the intense cruelty
of its expression. If ever proof were needed that the whole is greater than
the sum of its parts, it could be found in the organized persecutions of this
century. In street gangs and fraternities, in political oppression and tribal
warfare, and in the administration of the "final solution" (the extermination
of the Jewish people), group action has immeasurably magnified the power
of individual sadism.

Individual group members function in a recursive relationship with the
group as a whole; that is, as members choose groups and their own places
within them, in accordance with personal needs and motivations, group systems "assign" role functions to each member in accordance with current
group goals. As members work to achieve their own and the group's goals,
their mutual support empowers and also changes them.[2] That is the dynamic
meaning of "strength in numbers." Power is intoxicating, the more so when
it is enhanced by a feeling of security: security based, on the one hand, in
the unity and enchantment with one's fellows, and on the other hand, on

an idealization of the leader.[3] The reassuring power shared in the group and the comforting cohesion of fellowship are accompanied by the fear of being ostracized: ceasing to be one of "us" and becoming one of "them"—the others, out in the cold. Idealization of the leader implicitly devalues the members, who experience themselves as less in direct proportion to their overvaluation of the leader. From this it follows that members set aside their personal values in deference to group values promulgated by the leader.[4] Is it any wonder, then, that so many German citizens—by tradition molded to an authoritarian familial, national, and religious pattern—became "Hitler's Willing Executioners"?[5] Germans strove to achieve group ideals whilst also expressing personal fears and animosities, bolstered by the full power of the group intensifying personal sadism.

It is natural for the Hutu and the Tutsi tribes, the Croats and the Serbs, the Slavs and the Czechs, the Moslems and the Christians, the Amerindians and Caucasians to define their separate groups, banding together to protect their ideals, to empower themselves and their leaders in the full belief that they *are* right and that they *have* the right. The boundaries around each community have been drawn. Goodness is perceived to reside within, evil to belong outside. These boundaries are almost impermeable, and any communication across them threatens the purity of the ingroup with contamination by "evil" from the outgroup. And with this, humanity has divided itself into quasi-angels and devils—thereby justifying their scapegoating and torturing of the designated "devils," "vermin," "infidels," and "exploiters."

The pleasure of relieving oneself of fears and anger with the approval of the group, coupled with a conviction that such outrageous behavior promotes the common weal, reinforces both individual and group sadism. As Robert Prince put it, "One murder and a little blood just doesn't do it anymore."[6] However, social systems (families, clans, tribes, nations, and small groups)can also exert a degree of control over individual and collective expressions of hostile impulses. The great difficulty of containing hostile impulses rests in the natural fear of not getting enough—amplified into greed. And much of the power of the group over the individual derives from the human need for acceptance—which translates into being "good" by conforming. Compliance with group norms and similarity among group members are the conditions of acceptance, based on the (presumptive) operation of the "selfish gene" and "meme."[7]

While fear, and sometimes anger, are responses to *difference*, human empathy is an emotional response to a perceived *similarity*—the internal echo of another's condition. Accommodating oneself simultaneously to difference and similarity is the prerequisite for maintaining empathy for others in the context of restraining one's own sadistic acting-out of fear and anger. Given that the rewards for restraint and empathy usually are not immediate and, therefore, not as reinforcing as the relief obtained from discharging feelings, how can we hope to overcome "the dark impulses that lurk in the far regions of the soul, everywhere"?[8]

Today's potential for mass destruction threatens not only the groups at war, but also endangers humanity as a whole. Splitting the ingroup from the outgroup, the "good-us" from the "bad-you," is no longer self-preservative. Uncontrolled, unmodulated hostile aggression expressed with modern weaponry puts everyone's survival at risk. In other words, the probability of humanity's annihilation as a result of the instinctual protection of a family or tribal gene, or a national or societal "meme," is greater than the possibility of extinction by dilution of the gene-pool or the obliteration of a culture.[9] Freud was correct in recognizing that civilized man might overcome his instinctual aggression; he was far too optimistic in thinking that cognitive and moral processes alone would achieve that aim. Yes, cognition is involved: a *recognition* of the realistic *fear of annihilation* by modern warfare and oppression. Ultimately, however, we have to fight fire with fire, to rely on our primitive instincts. The impulse to aggress must be controlled by the instinct to survive, and the fear of annihilation likewise recognized and contained within each of us and within each group—not displaced[10] and enacted viciously against another—if anyone is to survive.

If the human power to act is magnified in groups, so is the potential to contain fear and hostility—as well as to restrain hostile enactments. Of course, group ideals, goals, and leadership are all important in determining the course traveled. And individual members—of families, clans, tribes, and nations—have much to learn about "sublimating"[11] their aggressive energies, into negotiating skills, for example. Is it possible? I have heard it said that "It takes two to keep the peace and only one to make war." Street-wise teenagers are certain that fists and weapons—not talk or walking away—will save their lives. On the other hand, after a couple of protected, precocious three-year olds were told to stop hitting each other, one of them stopped, thought, and declared to his friend, "We can disagree and still love each other." Which path will be taken?

The chapters in this book have described some effects on children of the trauma inflicted by societally organized hostility and persecution. The traumatic consequences of physical and verbal abuse in families are no less severe, lasting, or costly. The resulting painful memories, enervating apprehensiveness, and constricting self-consciousness are often quite invisible to outside observers, yet restrain even apparently well-adjusted survivors from fully potentiating their talents. The direct and transmitted effects of the trauma of oppression, prejudice, and untimely, forced separation from parents afflict not just the survivor, but generations. Jucovy's survivor in the barber shop, Judith Kestenberg's *Kindertransport* refugees, Godorowski's *muselman*, Milton Kestenberg's case of the mute husband, Kahn's and Fogelman's children with confused identities, Scheffel-Baars' ailments, Fried's and Valent's now-aging survivors who continue struggling to integrate their pasts, and even the Germans who still shudder when reflecting on their unstable lives—all are the victims of these organized "dark impulses." In one way or another, they have faced their experiences and were willing to speak of them. Most of the victims managed to heal themselves sufficiently to function in the world. They work, find partners, and raise families. In short, they cope. So did innumerable others who still decline to speak of their past, who try hard not to think of horrors, and strenuously avoid telling their children—communicating instead through silence. Although survivors may live a "normal" life like "everyone else," deep within them, the encapsulated poison may continue to corrode body and spirit.[12] They suffer from a variety of physical, psychosomatic, and psychological symptoms. Black moods becloud their lives.

The mere fact of surviving persecution is attributed by many of the oppressed to sheer luck. Psychologists and sociologists believe that, beyond luck, the pretraumatic personality and social supports are to be credited. For example, those ascribing their survival to "luck" tend to be resigned and despairing, and find it difficult to "give any sense or purpose to their lives." Others believe that their personal discipline, self-control, and social skills were significant in helping them to survive. Personality attributes such as "cunning maneuvering and skillful adaptation to the mentality of the guards . . . could get [the persecutee] assigned to perform easier types of work" and perhaps assigned to kitchen duties where food could be obtained. However, an isolated prisoner could not gain a foothold, as was the case for a German Jew assigned to a barracks with only Ukrainian prisoners. In this alien environment "he rapidly lost weight and died."[13]

Group power is not confined to the management of aggression; it extends to "social support and emotional involvements" facilitated by group cohesion, which is critical for survival.[14] Research shows that social support reduces the anxiety in youngsters exposed to military ground- and air-attacks. An Israeli study of children and adolescents living in "exposed" environments—kibbutzim ("socialist collectives characterized by a high degree of community organization . . . [and] communal rearing of children"), moshavim (agricultural cooperative, private enterprise communities where children are reared at home), and development towns (characterized by "a lower level of community organization and a weaker ideological commitment")—revealed "less personal anxiety and less behavior disturbance" and fewer concomitant symptoms among kibbutz members. This was attributed to the cohesive structure of the kibbutz: its "close-knit and ideologically committed group" and well-adapted adults who "serve as good role models" generally and "in stressful situations."[15]

The support of the parental relationship is crucial for young children. This was vividly demonstrated by the children who (unlike the "separated" children) showed "no signs of traumatic shock . . . [while] in the care of their own mothers or a familiar mother substitute" during the German bombings of Great Britain in World War II. Indeed, London children were reportedly more upset by evacuation than they were by the Blitz, and the war was less significant to them when it "only" threatened their lives, but it became "enormously significant the moment it breaks up family life."[16]

Family relationships continue to be extremely important even for older children and adolescents. One survivor was deported together with his parents from Germany to a French internment camp. Men and women were separated and, at age fifteen, he lived in the men's section with his father. His father was selected to be barracks chief and was, therefore, entitled to a separate room, which he shared with his son. After some time, the father was transferred out of the camp while his son, who remained alone, had to vacate the room and move to what was called the "rabbit warren," a large space with double-decker bunks in the center of the barracks. The young man recalls feeling utterly lost and dejected without his father. He wandered about aimlessly and was not sufficiently focused to hide when the Germans came to round up a complement of men to be assigned to forced labor at a different location. Once there, the stiff discipline, the back-breaking work, and the danger of being shot by the Germans aroused him out of his depressive stupor. Soon he contracted hepatitis and survived only as a result of a series of fortuitous events, one involving an SS officer who appeared at a critical juncture and secretly came to his aid. Finally, he found the strength to tell an audacious lie during a life-threatening moment. Weeks later, the laborers were returned to the internment camp, where they remained a cohesive group, supporting each other sufficiently so that the adolescent was prevented from relapsing into his depression. Years later, when asked to what he attributes his survival, he answered "Luck!" Yes, he had some luck, some of it in the form of social support. It was luck that he was at home when his family was picked up for deportation and that for a while in the camp he had the benefit of his father's protection; it was luck again that a compassionate person from among the oppressors happened to be near when he needed protection; and it was lucky that he was returned to the original camp in the company of his peers. But, in the final analysis, the supportive emotional and social involvements sustained him sufficiently to prevent him from succumbing to the debilitating forces of disease and from yielding to the passivity of the *muselman*.

Scheffel-Baars, too, was comforted by her social involvements. Like the adolescent boy in the concentration camp, she found help from some unlikely sources: her initiative in publicly confessing to her Nazi-collaborator father's guilt was rewarded by the response of the good quasi-father—another victim, a Jew in Israel, who helped her to make peace with her Nazi father. A trusting relationship with her pastor and her husband's support have enabled her to achieve a semblance of internal tranquility.

The Swedish schools opened for child and adolescent survivors immediately after the war, and the Café 84 in Stockholm, as well as the survivor groups of Australia, have also provided healing social support and emotional connections. In contrast, East Germans suffered anguish after the collapse of the communist state precisely because they lacked the supportive social structures. No patterns for initiating groups (outside of the politically-mandated organizations) had been established. Indeed, the pervasive mistrust and suspicion made any but the most superficial and stylized group activities all but impossible. Religion had been devalued, if not totally outlawed by communism, so that only occasionally would a parishioner seek personal comfort from a priest or perhaps from an inner connection to God. But supportive cohesion among a community of parishioners was beyond the realm of experience in communist East Germany. Only when this regime began to crumble did protesters find sufficient courage to risk banding together in order to empower themselves and each other. It was then that the churches became meeting places—but by no means always safe places, since many pastors violated the confidentiality to which they were bound by their vocation: They acted as informers for the Communist Party and the state.

There is little doubt that the stress imposed by the agony of the extermination camps, the limitless horrors of genocide, and the paranoia induced by totalitarian societies can override even a normal pretraumatic personality. Later re-experiencing (in contrast to recalling) of the traumatic experience is a manifestation of a failure of symbolization and integration. This cognitive deterioration might be explained by constricted functioning, perhaps due to regression to earlier developmental levels in response to extreme stress. There is also evidence that the great fluctuations in vulnerability both during and after incarceration are related to the pretraumatic personality. These are the "strands of influence."[17] One survivor had attributed his sensitivity and suspicion, his irritability and depressed moods to his suffering as a Jewish schoolboy (taunted and attacked by gentile schoolmates), compounded by the subsequent concentration-camp experience. In the course of psychotherapy he became aware that he had had bouts of depression even as a young boy and sad feelings as early as age five. A considerable depression torments him into his retirement age. To an outside observer it would seem that he has overcome his ordeals, healed, and leads a normal professional and family life. Yet he and his therapist know that the Holocaust, prejudice, and persecution are in his consciousness—daily, hourly—intensifying the childhood depressive feelings that, like uninvited guests, have resided within him throughout the years of his life.

Much about people's varying ability to cope despite adversity is still a mystery, though it appears to have its foundation in genetically-determined temperamental factors, including "high intelligence, physical resilience, and capacity for rapid and effective physical learning."[18] These attributes may help a survivor of social trauma to defend against an unacknowledged sense of weakness or shame and to go on with life despite feelings of rejection. However, true "invulnerability" is not defensive.[19] It manifests itself as "resiliency" in the face of life demands, and requires a full integration of personal feelings and past experiences; this leads, then, toward an authentic, stable sense of identity.

An integrated individual, equipped with resiliency and stability, is prepared to be empathetic even with strangers and is less vulnerable to capitulation to a leader and far less likely to act-out hostile impulses. The task for mental health professionals, educators, politicians, cultural leaders, and for the society at large is to devise supportive social structures on which parents can depend, so that they, in turn, will be enabled to create a nontraumatic climate of acceptance, respect, and "emotional involvement." These are the conditions permitting a benign dependence of children on adults, promoting an expansion of a child's psyche, including full cognitive development in the direction of symbolization and sublimation.

NOTES

1. William Clinton, Second Inaugural Address, Transcript of President Clinton's Second Inaugural Address to the Nation, *New York Times*, January 21, 1997.

2. Helen Durkin, "Analytic Group Therapy and General Systems Theory," in *Progress in Group and Family Therapy*, ed. C. Sager and H. Kaplan (New York: Bruner Mazel, 1972); Yvonne Agazarian, "Theory of the Invisible Group Applied to Individual and Group-As-A-Whole Interpretations" *Group* 7, no. 2 (Summer 1983): 27–37.

3. Sigmund Freud, "Group Psychology and the Analysis of the Ego" (1921), in *The Standard Edition of the Complete Psychological Works of Sigmund Freud* (London: The Hogarth Press, 1955), 18:69–143.

4. Ibid.

5. Daniel J. Goldhagen, *Hitler's Willing Executioners* (New York: Alfred A. Knopf, 1996).

6. Robert Prince, chapter 2, this volume.

7. Richard Dawkins, *The Selfish Gene* (New York: Oxford University Press, 1976).

8. Clinton, "Second Inaugural Address."

9. Dawkins, *Selfish Gene*.

10. Heinz Hartman, "Notes on the Theory of Sublimation," *Psychoanalytic Study of the Child* 10 (1955): 9–29; Ernst Kris, "Neutralization and Sublimation," *Psychoanalytic Study of the Child* 10 (1955): 30–46.

11. Kris, "Neutralization and Sublimation."

12. Paul Matussek, *Internment in Concentration Camps and Its Consequences* (1971; New York: Springer Verlag, 1975).

13. L. Eitinger, "Concentration Camp Survivors in Norway and Israel," in *Uprooting and After*, ed. Maria Pfister-Amende and Charles Zwingman (New York: Springer Verlag, 1973) 15, 114, and 191, maintains that "People of average mentality are capable of carrying on despite mental stress situations which may not affect their mental health to any great extent, provided that their personal and environmental anchorage is kept intact, and that the stress situations do not persist for too long." Eitinger also states that "premorbid deviations [prior to the traumatic experiences] appear to play a certain part" in severe psychological disturbances.

14. Miles E. Simpson, "Societal Support and Education," in *Handbook on Stress and Anxiety*, ed. Irwin Kutash et al. (San Francisco: Jossey-Bass, 1980), 451–62, quote cited on 457.

15. Norman Milgram, "War Related Stress in Israeli Children and Youth," in *Handbook of Stress: Theoretical and Clinical Aspects*, ed. Leo Goldberger and Shlomo Breznitz (New York: Free Press, 1982), 658, 657.

16. Anna Freud and Dorothy Burlingham, *War and Children* (New York: Ernst Williard, 1943), 21, 37.

17. See Milton Jucovy, chapter 1, this volume.

18. Edwin C. Peck, "The Traits of True Invulnerabiliy and Posttraumatic Stress in Psychoanalyzed Men of Action," in *The Invulnerable Child*, ed. E. James Anthony and Bertram J. Cohler (New York: The Guilford Press, 1987), 357.

19. Anthony and Cohler, *The Invulnerable Child*.

Bibliographical Essay

Charlotte Kahn

Organized persecution and war, interpersonal violence in families and on the city streets, and natural catastrophes can all causes trauma in children as well as in adults. By now the data on posttraumatic stress is so extensive, and the Holocaust literature so vast, that the selection here is perforce extremely limited. The references below will deal only with the social traumas (in contrast to the natural catastrophes).

For an exploration of poverty, homelessness, social, racial and sexual discrimination, seen as culturally supported maltreatment, and the familial contexts of child abuse, one might turn to John N. Briere, *Child Abuse Trauma: Theory and Treatment of the Lasting Effects* (Newbury Park, Calif.: Sage Publications, 1992). The long-term psychological impact of social abuse is discussed in detail, including posttraumatic stress, cognitive, relational, and emotional disturbances. One-half of the book is devoted to the philosophy and process of treating traumatized individuals. The traumatic Vietnam experience and its aftermath is presented in very personal terms through the images, feelings, and voices of the veterans who participate in "rap-groups" by Robert J. Lifton, *Home from the War* (New York: Simon and Schuster, 1973). Michael Norman, "The Hollow Man," *New York Times Magazine* (May 26, 1996) 54, also attests to the emotionally eviscerating aftereffects of war. See also Michael Norman, *These Good Men* (New York: Pocket Books, 1991).

Another detailed, personal account of socially organized trauma is that of Jack Werber with William B. Helmreich, *Saving the Children: Diary of a Buchenwald Survivor and Rescuer* (New Brunswick, N.J.: Transaction Publishers, 1997). Werber records his memories of the unbearably hard work, the hunger and cold, and the activities of the Underground, of collaborators, and of traitors in the Buchenwald concentration camp. When Werber had reached his nadir subsequent to learning of the death of his wife and infant daughter, 700 children were brought into the concentration camp. His attempts to save them saved him; keeping up the despairing children's hope for the future kept him alive to live his future.

While social psychologists can delineate certain conditions leading to oppression, and historians can point to the events immediately preceding a war, the psychological determinants of war are not at all clear. Ervin Staub postulates several preconditions for the Holocaust, such as a homogeneous population with a strong in-group spirit, a negative evaluation of subgroups, a sense of superiority, and devotion to lawfulness. Added to these conditions are a focus on and compartmentalization of goals, especially when the goals might conflict with values. The temptation to submit to a visionary authority is strong, and reinforcing propaganda and self-persuasion affect even the bystanders, who then refrain from intervening. Ervin Staub, *The Roots of Evil: The Origins of Genocide and Other Group Violence* (Cambridge: Cambridge University Press, 1989). Separate chapters are devoted to the conditions of the Turkish genocide of the Armenians, the Nazi Holocaust, Cambodia, and Argentina. Five antidotes to genocide and war are discussed, including child rearing methods.

"Why War?" (1933) is the question asked by Albert Einstein of Sigmund Freud. See *The Complete Psychological Works of Sigmund Freud*, ed. James Strachey (London: The Hogarth Press, 1964), 22: 197–215. This question is revisited by the contributors to Betty Glad, ed., *The Psychological Dimensions of War* (Newbury Park, Calif.: Sage Publications, 1990). In this book, biological roots, attraction to destruction, and learning are considered as possible causes for the decision to wage war. Five conditions sufficient to impute genocide are listed in Eric Marcusen and David Kopf, *The Holocaust and Strategic Bombing: Genocide and Total War in the Twentieth Century* (Boulder, Colo.: Westview Press, 1995). The authors wonder whether strategic bombing of civilian populations is genocidal. They consider the similarities and differences between the Holocaust and strategic bombing.

What of the fate of the survivors and their offspring? Rabinowitz writes the stories of the post–World War II immigrants she interviewed. Often using their vernacular of the English language, she manages to depict the personalities with all their sorrows, ambivalences, ambitions, and surprising successes. Included in the book is a chapter on the deportation proceedings of a female Vice-Kommandant of the Maidenek concentration camp; survivors living in America testified. Dorothy Rabinowitz, *New Lives: Survivors of the Holocaust Living in America* (New York: Avon, 1976). Helen Epstein, daughter of Holocaust survivors, felt she had dangerous things buried deep inside her in an iron box. The box was her vault to store her deceased family's history. Her book is comprised of the accounts of others like her: children of Holocaust survivors who were affected by their parents' lingering memories of trauma and loss. Helen Epstein, *Children of the Holocaust* (Toronto: Bantam Books, 1980). In another set of biographical accounts based on interviews, twenty-three photographs help to tell the history of the erstwhile child survivors of Terezin and Auschwitz who were sent to Lingfield, England, in 1945, to live in a group home under the care of Alice Goldberger. Sarah Moskovitz, *Love Despite Hate: Child Survivors of the Holocaust and their Adult Lives* (New York: Schocken Books, 1983).

Those interested in an emphasis on ethnocultural variations, including gender, might turn to Anthony J. Marsell, Matthew J. Friedman, Ellen T. Gerrity, and Raymond M. Scurfield, eds., *Ethnocultural Aspects of Posttraumatic Stress Disorder: Issues, Research, and Clinical Applications* (Washington, D.C.: American Psychological Association, 1996). The book is encyclopedic in scope and provides long reference lists at the conclusion of each chapter. It presents a synthesis of concepts and extensive empirical information on the posttraumatic syndrome and its treatment. In the course of treating trauma victims, therapists can be vicariously traumatized in various ways. This occurs as a result of their empathic engagement with their patients in the course of psychological/psychoanalytic treatment. The traumatized patients' tendency to communicate memories nonverbally, somatically, and with anxiety, coupled with the therapists' cumulative countertransferential responses, constitutes a danger to therapists and the therapy process. Laurie Ann Pearlman and Karen Saakvitne, *Trauma and the Therapist* (New York: W. W. Norton, 1995). This book focuses almost entirely on the trauma of childhood sexual abuse.

Two authors present parallel pedagogical and clinical phenomena in a book alternating literary and clinical perspectives in their search for the clash between violence and culture. As instructor of a class that becomes unexpectedly disoriented by reading a set of testimonials and viewing videotaped autobiographical reports of the Holocaust, Felman becomes aware of the power of the material and of her greater responsibility in teaching. The intense reactions of her students are documented with excerpts from their essays, which express new insights into their own history and personal dynamics. Laub contributes her psychiatric perspective. Shoshana Felman and Dori Laub, *Testimony: Crises of Witnessing in Literature, Psychoanalysis, and History* (New York: Routledge, 1992).

Grappling with a moral dilemma, Simon Wiesenthal retells the story told him by a wounded, dying *SS* man who has shot Jews, including a young child. The German asks Wiesenthal, the Jew, for forgiveness. Perplexed, the author submits the German's story to a symposium of more than thirty philosophers, clergy, and writers, inquiring what they would have done. This constitutes the second half of the book. Simon Wiesenthal, *The Sunflower* (Paris: Opera Mundi, 1969). The symposium members' thought-provoking responses and Wiesenthal's solution to his dilemma might motivate some readers to conduct their own moral introspection.

Index

Abandonment, 103, 111, 113, 116, 172, 224
Accident proneness, 171
Adolescents, 33–37, 41 n.49, 235
Affect disorders, 63. 189. *See also* Relationships
Aggression: by communities, 13; by individuals, 11–12
Aggressiveness, 119
Aggressor, identification with, 35, 40 n.37, 41 n.49, 103
Air raids, 197–99
Albert, King of Belgium, 228
Alexithymia, 63, 189. *See also* Relationships
Aloneness, 141–42
Altruism, 64
American Jewish Committee, 98
American Joint Distribution Committee, 27
Anger, of child Holocaust survivors, 61, 116
Anhedonia, 63
Anniversary reactions, 16
Antall, J., 100–101 n.9
Antisemitism: in Czechoslovakia, 98–99; and German Jews, 162–64; history of, 21–22; in Holland, 227; in Hun-

gary, 16, 90–101; in Poland, 98–99, 143; in Sweden, 174; types of, 20–21
Anxiety, 3, 20, 31, 79
Apathy, 112
Apocalyptic phenomena, 23–24, 38 n.16, 39 n.17
Appelfeld, Aharon, 26
Arabs, in Eastern Europe, 98
Arlow, Jacob, 38 n.10
Armenians, 44
Assertiveness, 12
Association of Child Survivors (Poland), 143
Australia, 106, 188–94

Barbers, 33–34
Bar-On, Dan, 124
Barzun, Jacques, 45
Beatrix, Queen of the Netherlands, 228
Bedwetting, 114
Beilis, Mendel, 22, 38 n.9
Bernadotte, Count Folke, 176
Bettelheim, Bruno, 48–49
Bienstock, Bonnie, 88
Birth rate, 50
Blacks, in Eastern Europe, 98
Blame, for victim, 51

About the Editors
and Contributors

EVA FOGELMAN is a psychologist in private practice. She is codirector of psychotherapy with Generations of the Holocaust and Related Traumas, Training Institute for Mental Health and a senior research fellow at the Center for Social Research, CUNY Graduate Center.

HEDI FRIED is a psychologist in Stockholm, Sweden, where she is also director of Café 84, a gathering place for Holocaust survivors.

KAZIMIERZ GODOROWSKI, Ph.D., wrote his dissertation on *Psychology and Psychopathology of the Nazi Concentration Camps* and published over seventy articles on human life under extreme conditions. Before his retirement he worked at the Mental Clinics Zabki-Drewnica in Warsaw and lectured on diagnostic methods in psychiatry and forensic psychology in the Institute of Psychology at the Theological Academy in Warsaw. During World War II he was a soldier of resistance in the Home Army (Polish Resistance group) until arrested by the Gestapo and sent to the Gross Rozen concentration camp.

LITZI HART is a physiotherapist and Feldenkrais practitioner in Sydney, Australia.

MILTON JUCOVY, M.D., is a psychoanalyst in Great Neck, New York, training and supervising analyst at the New York Psychoanalytic Institute, and a founding chairman of the Group for the Psychoanalytic Exploration of the Effects of the Holocaust on the Second Generation. He is co-editor of *Generations of the Holocaust* (1982).

CHARLOTTE KAHN, Ed.D., is a psychoanalyst and family therapist. She has served on the faculties of college, graduate, and postgraduate institutions since 1966. She is currently adjunct associate professor in the Department of Psychology, City College of the City University of New York. She has served on the faculties of the New Jersey Institute of Psychoanalysis and Psychotherapy, the National Psychological Association for Psychoanalysis, and has appeared on radio and television in connection with her family therapy work. Her articles have appeared in *Psychoanalytic Study of the Child, Psychoanalytic Review,* and *The Journal of Psychohistory,* she is a contributor to *Children During the Nazi Reign: Psychological Perspectives on the Interview Process* (Praeger, 1994). She is a member of the editorial board of the *Psychoanalytic Review* and is co-editor of *Immigration: Personal Narrative, Psychological Analysis* (1997).

JUDITH S. KESTENBERG, M.D., a psychoanalyst, is a supervising and training analyst emeritus for adults and children at New York University Psychoanalytic Institute and is on the psychiatric staff of Long Island Jewish Medical Center in New Hyde Park, N.Y. She is one of the founders and organizers and the director of Child Development Research, which uses the Kestenberg Movement Profile (KMP) for Developmental Assessment. She is co-director and project director of the International Study of Organized Persecution of Children, now affiliated with Tel-Aviv University. She is also the founder of the Group for the Psychoanalytic Study of the Effect of the Holocaust on the Second Generation. Among Dr. Kestenberg's professional contributions to the literature are *Children and Parents* (1975), *The Role of Movement Patterns in Development, Vol. I* (1977), and *The Role of Movement Patterns in Development, Vol. II* (1979). She is the author of numerous articles and a main contributor to *Generations of the Holocaust,* edited by Martin S. Bergmann and Milton E. Jucovy (1982), as well as co-editor with Dr. Eva Fogelman of *Children During the Nazi Reign: Psychological Perspectives on the Interview Process* (Praeger, 1994).

MILTON KESTENBERG, Esq., an attorney, co-founder of the Group for Psychoanalytic Study of Psychological Effects on the Second Generation, and co-founder of the International Study of Organized Persecution of Children, is deceased.

JUDIT MÉSZÁROS, Ph.D., is a psychoanalytic psychotherapist in Budapest, Hungary. She is affiliated with the Institute of National Medical Rehabilitation, teaches at the Postgraduate Medical University of Budapest, and is on the editorial board of the journal *Thalassa,* published in Hungary.

ROBERT PRINCE, Ph.D., a clinical psychologist in private practice, is on the faculty of the New York University Postdoctoral Program in Psychoanalysis and Psychotherapy. He has lectured extensively on the psychological effects of the Holocaust on the survivors and their families, on children of survivors, as well as on the impact of the Holocaust on identity. He is the author of *The Legacy of the Holocaust: Psychohistorical Themes in the Lives of Children of Survivors* (1985).

GONDA SCHEFFEL-BAARS, M.A., a history teacher of adults in Amsterdam, Holland, has written articles about Dutch collaborators and their children.

PAUL VALENT, M.D., a child survivor, is author of *Child Survivors: Adults Living with Childhood Trauma* (1994). He is a psychiatrist in private practice in Melbourne, Australia, and is affiliated with Monash University Medical Centre, Accident and Emergency Department, and the Australian Society for Traumatic Stress Studies. He is a member of the Child Survivors of the Holocaust Group in Melbourne.

NIKOLA VOLF, M.D., Ph.D., professor of Neuropsychiatry, Belgrade University, and head of the Neuropsychiatric Department, Belgrade City Hospital (retired), has published close to 120 professional articles. His father, a Yugoslavian-Jewish pediatrician, survived several concentration camps; his mother was killed in Auschwitz. During World War II he served in the Yugoslav army and as a medical assistant in the Jewish Hospital in Budapest, Hungary. He survived fourteen months in a forced labor unit.

ISBN 0-275-96261-X

EAN

HARDCOVER BAR CODE

90000>